CRACKING THE DIET CODE

The ultimate guide to understanding your body and responding with the right nutrition

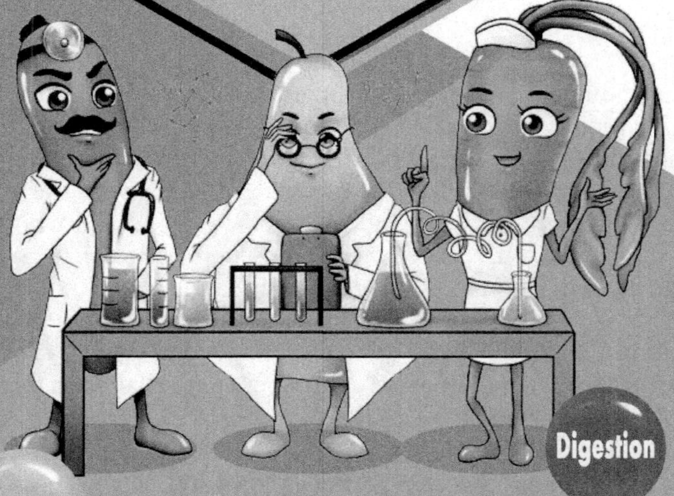

ALISON COWELL

To my gorgeous grandchildren Jack, Jessica and Maverick (and those I may yet meet!), may you always be healthy and happy.

Published by Goldcrest Books International Ltd
Design and Typeset by Tiger Media
Cover artwork and illustrations by Sophie Blokker

www.goldcrestbooks.com

publish@goldcrestbooks.com

ISBN: 978-1-913719-73-9

Contents

Preface		v
Introduction		vii
Part 1 The Digestive System – Your Engine		11
Chapter 1	Your Digestive Team	13
Chapter 2	Tips to Support Overall Digestive Health	22
Chapter 3	Probiotics	27
Chapter 4	The Perfect Poo!	32
Chapter 5	Signs of Nutrient Deficiencies	34
Chapter 6	Food Intolerances	40
Chapter 7	The Microbiome and Our Gut–Brain Axis	50
Part 2 Natural Remedies for Common Health Issues		53
Chapter 1	Digestive Disorders	55
Chapter 2	Hormone-related Disorders	78
Chapter 3	Nervous System Disorders	94
Chapter 4	Skin and Hair Disorders	102
Chapter 5	Joint and Bone Disorders	116
Chapter 6	Blood and Circulatory Disorders	122
Chapter 7	Lung Disorders	130
Chapter 8	Pregnancy	132
Chapter 9	Immune System Disorders	134
Chapter 10	Chronic Fatigue Syndrome	141
Chapter 11	Cancer	146
Part 3 Medications, Supplements and Eating Well		149
Chapter 1	Medication and Food Conflicts	151
Chapter 2	Supplements	160
Chapter 3	Eating Well	170

And Finally...		**199**
Appendix 1	Tips for Weight Loss	**200**
Appendix 2	Understanding Thyroid Results	**204**
Appendix 3	Tyramine	**206**
Appendix 4	Meal Ideas to Fight Depression, Anxiety and Insomnia	**208**
Appendix 5	Salicylates	**210**
Appendix 6	Hints and Tips for Shift Workers	**214**
Appendix 7	Oestrogen Level Score Chart	**216**
Appendix 8	Pregnancy Trimesters	**218**
Appendix 9	Food and Symptom Diary	**220**
About Me		**222**
Acknowledgements		**224**
Index		**225**

Preface

When it comes to health and food, we are bombarded with information from many sources these days: friends, family, work colleagues, 'experts', TV documentaries, Google, social media, clever marketing and more, often with conflicting advice. No wonder we get so confused! Most are genuinely offering what they believe to be the best information, but we are all unique and what suits one person may not suit another. Most of us are aware of what 'healthy' food is, but what happens when we choose the healthy option and don't get the results we deserve? What if the fruit and vegetable choices we're making are working against us rather than for us?

At the time of writing, I've seen almost 11,000 individual clients in my clinics both in New Zealand and the UK. Every single one of them knew what a 'healthy' diet should be, yet here they were with elevated cholesterol, thyroid problems, digestive complaints, skin problems ... and so on. Not because they weren't doing their best, but because they didn't have the right knowledge to make the best choices for themselves.

Looking at facts, your body runs on cellular activity and every cell needs the correct nutrients in order to be able to function. Needs change with different stages of life, so it's important to ensure you are providing your system with the correct nutrients at each of these stages (for example, your teenage body requires different nutrients to that of your 60-year-old body).

Meanwhile, whilst there is a wealth of information on food, what is hardly ever acknowledged is the system that breaks down that food – your digestive system. You could have the most perfect diet, but if you have digestive issues or food intolerances, they become barriers that interfere with nutrients reaching your cells. Combine that with the side-effects of medications, and you could unwittingly be creating many of the health issues you are seeking to resolve.

I have written this book based on my own personal health experience and the knowledge gained from seeing thousands of clients in my clinics. I hope you find it informative and enlightening but, more than that, I hope it motivates you to make the right choices to invest in your current and future health.

Alison Cowell

Introduction

Knowledge–Choice–Consequence

For most things in life we follow the pattern of knowledge, choice and consequence. For instance, when choosing a new home, we know the area we want to go to, we know how much money we have to spend and we make our choices based on that knowledge. The consequence is living in an area we like that is within our means. Holidays, insurances, cars, even relationships, all follow the knowledge–choice–consequence flow.

However, when it comes to health it seems we do everything back to front! We start with the consequence, the health issue: maybe it's the diagnosis of type 2 diabetes or a heart attack or a cancer scare, or whatever. That 'consequence' encourages us to choose what we might want to do about it and, for most of us, that choice is simply to go to the doctor. There's nothing wrong with that, but it's not the only choice you have.

The reason we tend to not look too much further is that we don't have enough knowledge – either about the condition that we have or about our own body's needs.

That's what this book is going to give you – the knowledge to make the right choices to have the health consequences you deserve!

Uniquely You

There is no one like you in the world – isn't that good to know! Despite over 7 billion people inhabiting this wonderful planet of ours, you are completely unique – even if you are an identical twin. You've become who you are as a result of many factors.

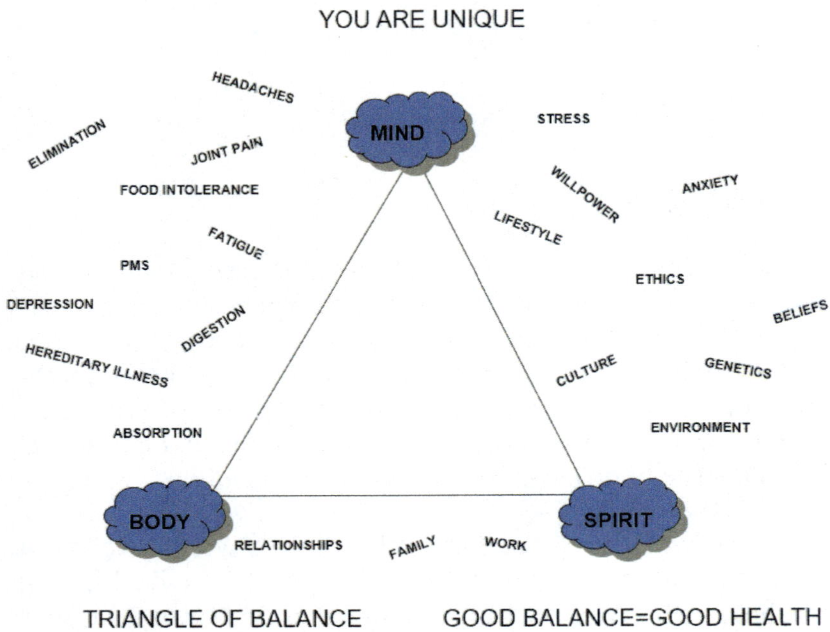

Our uniqueness means that our systems don't always respond in predictable ways, and when it comes to food and nutrition, that matters!

Engine and Fuel

Quite often in my health awareness seminars, I tell the story of the time that our friend Trevor put diesel in our lovely Daimler car instead of petrol. The results were catastrophic (both for the car and the friendship!) The point of telling this story is to highlight the fact that there was nothing wrong with the engine and nothing wrong with the fuel – they just didn't go together.

And so it is with our human bodies. Just because a food is 'healthy' doesn't mean it is right for your system. There are many reasons why this could be, including allergies or intolerances (there is a difference, as we'll discover later), poor digestive health, a conflict with medications, a conflict with a condition (for example, acidic foods like tomatoes can aggravate arthritic conditions), and so on.

We will be looking at the fuel (your food) throughout this book but, before that, we need to ensure the engine (your digestive system) is firing on all cylinders. It has the very important job of feeding all your cells so it's important to keep it healthy, because if it doesn't work very well, neither will you.

Part 1

The Digestive System – Your Engine

The digestive tracts inside us humans are the same today as they were when we first walked the Earth thousands of years ago. The functions of each organ are the same, the juices and enzymes they produce are the same, the way they break down food and eliminate waste is the same, even the way they react to foreign particles or 'invaders' is the same (and food intolerances could be classed as both!) However, as we have evolved and spread ourselves through different continents with different soils, different fruits and vegetables and, indeed, different meats and fish, our digestive systems have had to adapt quite radically.

One of the fundamental changes is the combinations of foods we eat. Thinking back, we would kill an animal, eat the meat from it and that would be it. We didn't run off and get a tree or a bush to eat with the meat protein. If there were no animals around, we would satisfy ourselves with the vegetation, leaves and shoots that were available. So, we didn't combine our food; proteins and carbohydrates were eaten at different times. Nowadays, things are different. We have an abundance of food ready at all times and we eat a mixture of them all at one time. If your digestive

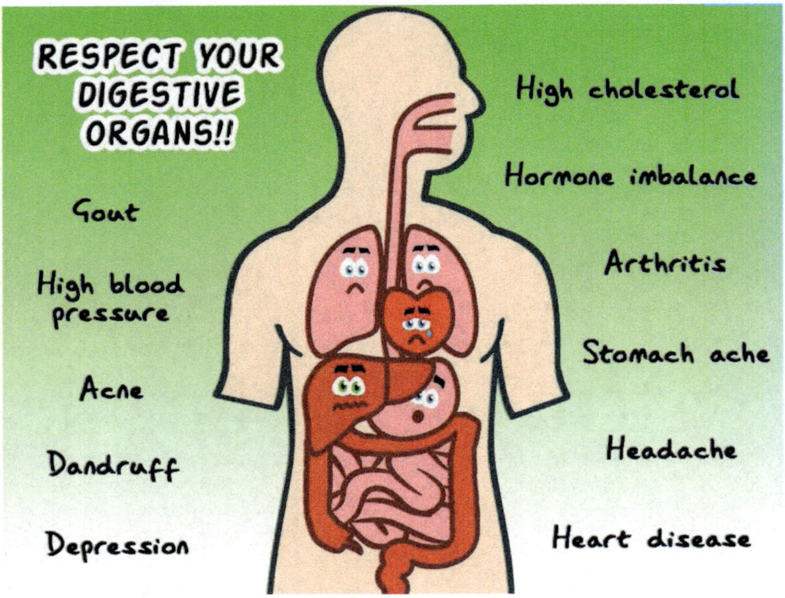

Illustration by Jeremy Woods.

system is robust and you have no issues (e.g. reflux, bloating, gas, etc.), then there's no problem combining your food groups. But if you do experience any digestive discomfort, then before you resort to medications or digestive aids, why not understand what's happening inside your body to see if you can address the cause, rather than treat the symptom? To do that, it helps to know what's going on internally.

Chapter 1

Your Digestive Team

There are a variety of wonderful systems working within your body, but many of us are oblivious to where they are and what they do. I remember when I first studied nutrition, I was in a class of 26 adult students. The tutor asked us where the spleen was. There was a moment of awkward silence as most of us gazed hard at our pens or brushed imaginary dust from our notebooks. Finally, one brave soul put up their hand and asked if it was "here", pointing randomly to the entire abdominal area in elaborate circles. No, it wasn't.

That episode brought home to me how ignorant I was to the systems and organs that were keeping me alive and healthy. As I learned more about them, I was (and remain) in awe of the incredible workings and interconnections of these amazing life-giving systems that we often so readily take for granted:

- **Digestive system**
- **Cardiovascular/circulatory system (the heart and blood vessels)**
- **Exocrine system (the skin, hair, nails and sweat)**
- **Muscular system/skeletal system (the muscles and bones)**
- **Nervous system (the link between the brain, muscle and nerve functions)**
- **Renal system/urinary system (the kidneys, bladder and urinary tract)**
- **Reproductive system (the ovaries, womb, testicles, etc.)**
- **Respiratory system (the lungs, trachea, pharynx, larynx, etc.)**
- **Sensory system (sensory receptors, neural pathways and parts of the brain involved in sensory perception).**

I have deliberately placed the digestive system at the top of the list as it is pivotal to your health. It literally is the engine feeding the cells that help make all the other systems work efficiently.

Whilst I am sure many of you will know quite a bit about what we perceive to be 'healthy' foods and 'superfoods' – what do you know about your digestive system, your amazing engine that processes them?

It's time to meet this incredible team.

Tongue

An average tongue is about 8 cm long. Together with your teeth and saliva, your tongue helps to break down the food in your mouth, pulping it ready to move forward through your digestive tract. There are taste buds on your tongue, clustered in four places, and they send receptors to your brain. This is when you might start pulling a face if you're not keen on a flavour or salivating more if you're loving it!

Many digestive issues arise simply because we are not chewing our food thoroughly. This is the only part of digestion that you have absolute control over and, as noted in Chapter 2 (page 22), there are no cutting tools inside you. Use your tongue and teeth well! The tongue is also an indicator of internal health (page 36).

Pharynx (throat)

Your pharynx (also part of the respiratory system) is a soft, cone-shaped, narrow tube that squeezes food down to your oesophagus when you swallow. It is about 12.5 cm long.

Oesophagus (the gullet)

This muscular tube connects your pharynx to your stomach. It's about 25 cm long and around 1.5 cm wide. Your oesophagus mixes your food with mucus and squeezes it down to your stomach. When the oesophagus is impaired, stomach acid may enter and contribute to reflux and indigestion. Too much air entering your system at this early stage of digestion will lead to a build-up of gas.

Stomach

Your stomach is about the size of your fist, but it can expand to accommodate a large meal or fluid intake.

Many foods are broken down with acidic stomach enzymes like hydrochloric acid and pepsin, and others are broken down with alkaline enzymes like ptyalin. When you eat foods together that require opposing enzymes (acid and alkaline), they neutralise each other in your stomach. This causes digestion to slow or stop altogether.

Signs of low stomach acid (hypochlorydia) include weak splitting fingernails. This is important to know considering more than half of over 60-year-olds have this condition! The symptoms of hypochlorhydria and hyperchlorhydria (high stomach acid) are similar. Many people are treated for high stomach acid when they actually have low stomach acid, so the treatments are often making the situation worse.

There are various tests you can do to determine how weak or strong your stomach acids are, including the baking soda test. First thing in the morning, before eating or drinking, mix ¼ teaspoon of baking soda in 4–6 fl oz of water. Drink the solution slowly (gulping could produce gas) and time how long it takes you to burp. If your stomach is producing adequate amounts of stomach acid, you'll burp within two to three minutes. Early and repeated burping may indicate high stomach acid, any burping after 3 minutes may indicate low stomach acids. You can try the test over three separate days.

Bowel

This tube-like organ starts at your stomach, ends at your anus and is made up of your large and small intestines. The 'small bowel' is the upper part of your intestine and takes nutrients from the food you eat. Your colon and rectum form your 'large bowel', which is located low in your pelvic floor. Ongoing pain or discomfort in this area should not be ignored as it can be a sign of inflammatory bowel conditions such as ulcerative colitis, Crohn's disease and diverticulitis.

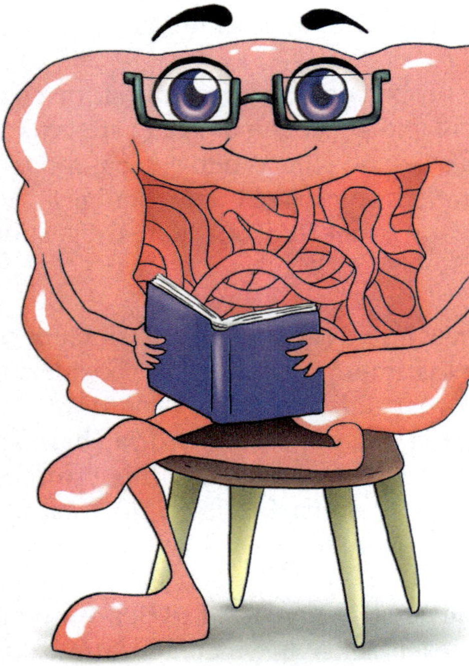

You can improve your bowel function by increasing the number of healthy bacteria and the amount of fibre in your diet. Fermented foods like kimchi, kombucha and sauerkraut have proven benefits to strengthen the bowel and improve overall digestive health. There are also many foods that help stimulate peristalsis (the muscle action required to help push food through your digestive tract) and the food-combining tips mentioned on page 13 will also be beneficial.

It will help your bowel function if you lean forward when on the toilet because our bodies work more effectively when we adopt a 'squat' position to expel waste.

Liver

This meaty organ is the second largest single organ in your body (the skin being the largest) and weighs around 2 kg. It is approximately 22 cm in diameter and 16 cm in height.

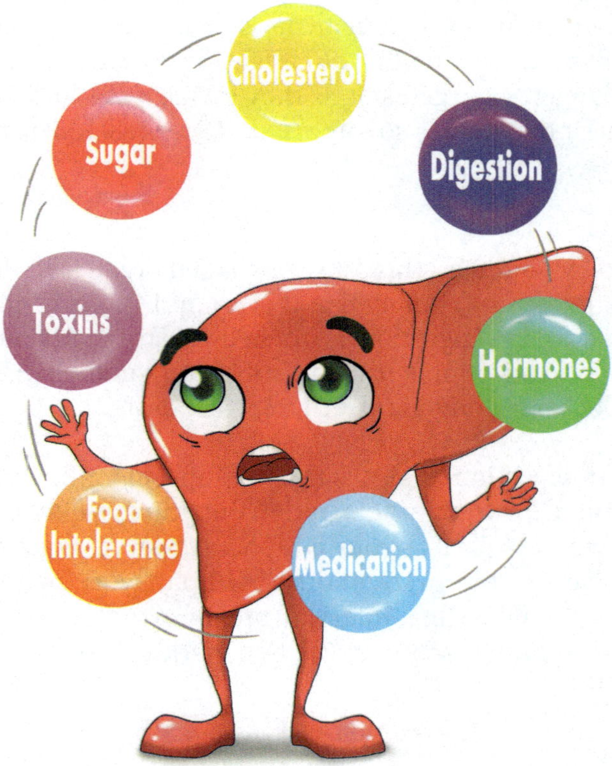

Your liver is responsible for over 500 different functions, making it one of the hardest-working organs in your body. It plays a role in detoxification, blood sugar regulation, production of bile, elimination of bad cholesterol and hormonal balance. In fact, conditions such as PMS; fibrocystic breast disease; ovarian cysts; uterine fibroids, and cancer of the breast, ovaries and uterus are associated with elevated oestrogen, which can be the result of the liver not breaking down oestrogen efficiently.

Gallbladder

This organ sits by your liver and measures 7–10 cm. It stores the bile acids produced by your liver, helps emulsify the fats and oils you eat and is essential to the processing of fat-soluble vitamins A, D, E and K. Bile also regulates the level of healthy bacteria in your system and helps stimulate peristalsis (the muscular action that pushes food through your digestive tract). It also helps destroy dangerous organisms as they invade your body which is why healthy bile flow is so important. (See Gallstones, page 58)

Spleen

Protected by your ribs, this sausage-shaped organ is in the upper far left part of your abdomen and is around 11 cm at its widest point. Its role in digestion is to help absorb nutrients from digested food in your small intestine and send them to cells throughout your body via your lymphatic system.

Other than digestion, it also acts as a filter, separating clean and unclean fluids in your system and maintaining the fluid balance in your body. As part of your lymphatic system, your spleen is also involved in the production of lymphocytes (white blood cells) that defend against infection and help the development of specific immunities. More on the lymphatic system on page 134

Pancreas

Your pancreas is part of your endocrine system (the system for producing most of the hormones in your body) but is important in the digestive process. It is approximately 15 cm long and sits behind your stomach. The pancreas produces hormones called insulin and glucagon. Insulin helps your blood cells absorb sugar from the food you eat and converts it into energy. If there is too much sugar in your diet, the pancreas is unable to make enough insulin and excess sugar gets into your bloodstream. On the other hand, if blood sugar levels are too low, glucagon is released. Either situation can result in type-2 diabetes if left unchecked.

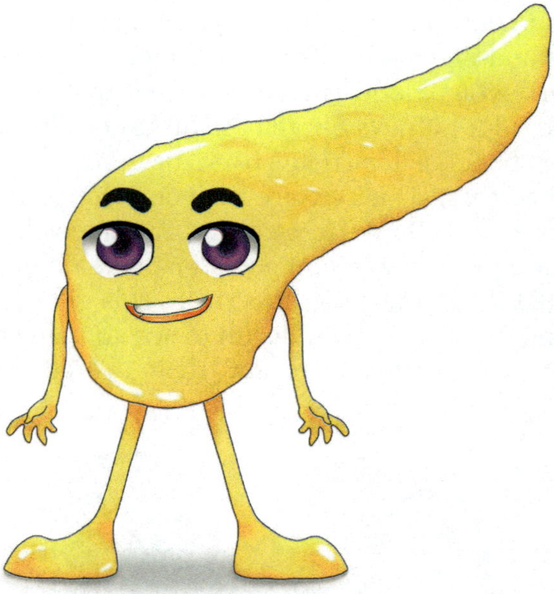

All carbohydrate foods are broken down into glucose (a type of sugar), and your brain uses this to function. I've seen so many clients who opted for a strict 'no-sugar' diet and who came to see me as they had 'fuzzy' heads and couldn't think straight. Some had also noticed a change in their mood and behaviour. That's not surprising, as there is a direct link between blood sugar balance and mood. The more uneven your blood sugar supply, the more uneven your mood. There's more on the role of the pancreas in the diabetes section starting on page 81.

Many women with polycystic ovary syndrome (PCOS) have insulin resistance, so it's worth getting your levels checked if you have a history of this condition.

Kidneys

Although not part of the digestive team, I've included the kidneys here because they support cells in the body that eliminate waste, including the digestive system. Located in the lower part of your back on either side of your spine, this pair of organs (each about the size of your fist) is busy every second of the day.

Every day your kidneys sift out approximately 4 pints of waste products and extra water from your blood. As a result of their hard work, your blood is free of toxins that could make you very sick. Your kidneys can tell the difference between harmful toxins and beneficial nutrients from the food you eat. They filter out the bad things, and ensure the good things are reabsorbed into your blood. Blood test results can show how well your kidneys are performing, and an estimated glomerular filtration rate (estGFR) shows how effectively this filtering process is happening. It has been wonderful to see so many of my clients improve their estGFR score and their overall wellbeing as a result.

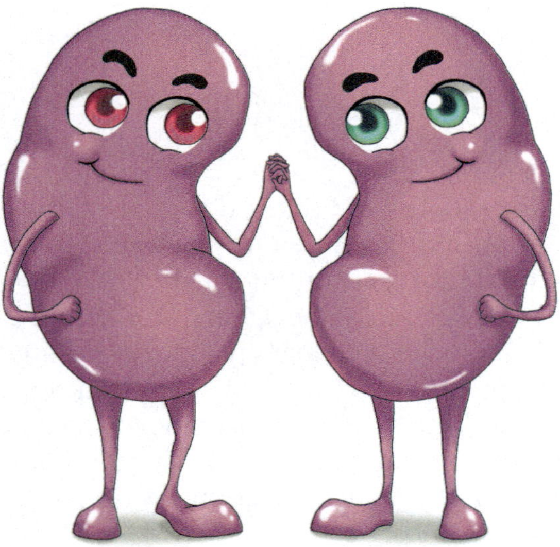

Creatinine is a waste product formed by the normal breakdown of muscle cells. Healthy kidneys take creatinine out of the blood and put it into the urine to be excreted. When the kidneys are not working well, creatinine builds up in the blood. Again, a blood test will reveal your levels and you can then target any aspect that needs to be addressed.

High blood pressure can damage the small blood vessels in your kidneys and that prevents them filtering waste efficiently. If kidney damage has occurred, then you need to eat low potassium foods such as garlic, berries, cranberries, onions and apples, and limit intake of high potassium foods such as bananas, potatoes, oranges, caffeine, chocolate, avocados and kiwi fruit.

The kidneys are also responsible for fluid, mineral, potassium and pH balance – so keep them happy!

Summary

Now you are familiar with your digestive organs. This lovely team is working every second of every day to keep all aspects of your health in tip-top condition.

In the next chapter I've provided some useful tips on how you can keep your digestive system working effectively because, as you'll find out later, when it doesn't work very well, neither do you.

Chapter 2

Tips to Support Overall Digestive Health

These simple tips neatly summarise some of the main points from the previous pages. You'll be familiar with most, I'm sure – but do you do them?!

If you're experiencing digestive issues, it may help if you take these on board to see the impact they can have. I've found that older digestive systems in particular respond very well, with conditions such as diverticulitis and reflux being greatly improved.

- **Take time to enjoy the aroma of your food and drink.**
  Why? Digestion begins with the sight and smell of food. Smell triggers saliva production, and saliva helps break down the particles of food in your mouth. Slow down and savour the experience!

- **Ensure you chew your food thoroughly before you swallow.**
  Why? Because you have no sharp teeth or cutting tools inside your digestive tract – if your teeth couldn't handle it, your insides will struggle. What isn't processed by your gastric juices will be stored as fat and/or toxic waste. Chewing also stimulates the production of stomach acid. The only part of digestion you have control over is chewing – so do a good job!

- **Avoid combining fruits with other food and do not have a fruit dessert until an hour after a meal.**
  Why? Because fruit is absorbed rapidly (within 30 minutes) and requires different digestive juices to that of your protein and carb main meal. Animal products contain toxic waste, together with fat and protein, and so take longer to digest than fruit.

- **Aid your digestion by eating proteins and carbs separately. You don't have to worry about planning separate meals. Rather, eat your vegetables first, then move on to your carbs (potatoes/rice, etc.) and finish with your protein (meat/fish, etc.)**
  Why? Food groups require different digestive enzymes and acids. For example, proteins need acid digestive juices and take 4 hours to reach the bowel, while carbs require alkaline juices and take 2 hours to reach the bowel. Most proteins digest in the stomach, whilst carbs digest in the small intestine, which is why they do not 'combine' well when eaten together.

- **Begin your evening meal with a few mouthfuls of raw food (e.g. salad, diced veg, coleslaw, etc.)**
  Why? To provide your system with living enzymes that will aid digestion and support your stomach acids. It will also help protect you from a condition known as 'digestive leukocytosis', which is where white blood cells (leukocytes) concentrate on aiding digestion rather than protecting you from viruses, etc.

- **Drink water throughout the day (avoid gulping it down in large quantities – just sip regularly).**
  Why? Water improves digestion, helps carry the nutrients round your body and flushes out toxins. The more you intake, the fuller you will feel and hunger pains will be reduced or even avoided.

- **Do not eat burnt food.**
  Why? Because burnt food can be hard to digest and it's carcinogenic. When barbecuing meat, cook slowly and evenly and do not have the coals directly underneath the meat.

- **Avoid any green discolouration in potatoes and chips.**
  Why? They contain toxins called glykoalkaloids that can seriously interfere with digestion. Avoid sprouted potatoes for the same reason.

- **Be aware of your portion sizes and don't overload your plate.**
  Why? Although your stomach can expand to deal with the extra load, it means it will have to work harder – as will all your other digestive organs. Small portions encourage better digestion, giving your system adequate time to process and absorb nutrients.

- **Buy fresh, preferably organic produce.**
  Why? Fresh – because food starts to lose its goodness as soon as it is picked or harvested. Organic – because it means the food (plant and animal) has been grown without the use of pesticides, additives, synthetic fertilisers or growth hormones – all of which build up in our systems when eaten. Fresh and organic products will also be free from harmful preservatives, additives and colourings, reducing the toxic load on your liver.

- **Avoid drinking when you eat – i.e. sip before and afterwards but not during your meal.**
  Why? Because it can upset your body's own natural digestive juices and cause gas and bloating.

- **Avoid having foods and drinks that are either very hot or very cold.**
  Why? Because you may cause damage to your digestive tract over time.

- **Rinse fruit and vegetables in a solution of apple cider vinegar and water.**
  Why? Plain water alone will not get rid of pesticides, and they can cause an array of health issues once ingested.

- **Add probiotics or fermented food to your daily intake.**
  Why? Healthy bacteria aid absorption of nutrients and can prevent many digestive issues arising.

- **Keep a food and symptom diary if you're experiencing ongoing digestive issues.**
  Why? It can help highlight specific foods or their combinations that your digestive system struggles with. See Appendix 9 on pages 220–221 for a template.

Tips for Eating Out

- Once you know the restaurant you are going to, contact them prior to arrival to let them know you have food intolerances and identify suitable alternatives.

- If having a drink, remember to sip before and after your meal but not while you are eating to aid digestion and avoid discomfort.

- Try to avoid eating any bread before your starter. Sensitivities to both yeast and wheat are quite common and can adversely affect your digestive system.

- Always choose melon for a starter if it's available. It's easy to digest and will not interfere with your protein and carb main meal. Failing that, other fruits for a starter are acceptable, preferably on their own because fruit doesn't mix well with other food. If fruit is not available as an option, choose a light soup.

- Main courses that have been baked, broiled, roasted, poached or steamed will be healthier and easier to digest than anything fried. Salads with fresh vegetables and light dressings will be better than salads with croutons, cheeses, meats and heavy dressings.

- Request sauces to be served separately.

- Chew slowly and thoroughly and don't feel obliged to clear your plate (restaurant portions can be on the large side!)

- Avoid having a fruit dessert, unless an hour has passed from your main meal, as it will not mix well on top of your protein and carb main meal.

- If you are going out for an evening meal and adhering to your circadian clock, try not to eat too late at night. If that can't be avoided, try to start eating later in the day, so you don't overactivate your digestive system (causing it to store undigested food as fat).

Chapter 3
Probiotics

We hear a lot about them, but what exactly are they? Clients often proudly announce they are having 'acidophilus yoghurt' without perhaps fully appreciating the impact that this particular strain of bacteria is having on their entire system.

Probiotics are amazing live microorganisms that are finally coming under a well-deserved spotlight.

Our 'microbiome' is the collection of healthy bacteria that reside in our gut (over one hundred trillion of them) and is often referred to as our second brain. Our two brains communicate via the vagus nerve, which connects them. This communication channel is known as the gut–brain axis and links biochemical signals between our gastrointestinal tract and our central nervous system. I've covered this in more detail on page 50–51.

Scientific research has been uncovering the microbiome's association with many body functions and systems, including our immunity, skin, mental health and yes, even our weight. I am convinced that there will eventually be a link with a particular species and the Covid19 virus.

In my clinics, I have witnessed amazing transformations in clients who have regularly taken the correct probiotic for their needs. Although most sound like spells from a Harry Potter novel, luckily you don't have to pronounce them! They will be clearly listed on the back of the products you are buying.

The Lactobacillus species is the most abundant friendly bacteria and particularly helpful for those who have an issue with lactose intolerance. They are responsible for producing lactase, the enzyme required to break down lactose (the sugar in milk). Another prolific strain is *Bifidobacteria*.

My particular favourites include:

Lactobacillus acidophilus: perhaps the most familiar of all the species, they colonise most densely in the small intestine and help absorption of nutrients. They can help prevent/relieve symptoms of both diahorrea and constipation and have also been shown to support urinary and vaginal health.

Lactobacillus helveticus: a close second to the *rhamnosus* below, I am amazed by the power of this magnificent species, which can aid emotional and mental wellbeing. So many of my clients were able to avoid antidepressants by regular intake of probiotics containing this strain (together with *Bifidobacterium longum*).

Lactobacillus plantarum: present in saliva and also in fermented foods, it produces hydrogen peroxide, which can help kill harmful bacteria in food. It has been shown to relieve the symptoms of IBS. *Plantarum* is also particularly effective in supporting the immune system.

Lactobacillus rhamnosus: ok, I've got to admit, this wonderful little species is right at the top of my list as I have seen many people respond so well with it. Apart from aiding with digestion (it's well known to prevent traveller's diarrhoea), supporting vaginal health and helping with mood disorders, it has an incredible effect on skin. Honestly, from common conditions such as acne and eczema to the more challenging psoriasis and Grover's disease, I have watched 'hopeless' cases respond quite dramatically.

Lactobacillus salivarius: this is great for supporting oral health and boosting the immune system.

Lactobacillus reuteri: a good all-rounder that supports oral health, immunity and digestion.

Lactobacillus paracasei: very effective for those suffering with grass pollen allergies

Bifidobacterium lactis 420: for controlling body fat, balancing glucose levels, promoting nutrient absorption and aiding weight loss.

Bifidobacterium bifidum: when combined with *Streptococcus thermophilus* or *Bifidobacterium Bb12* it can help prevent rotoviral diarrhoea in children.

Also, not to be forgotten, is **Butyric Acid (Butyrate)**. It is a short-chain fatty acid produced by gut bacteria from undigested plant fibre. The more you have, the less likely you are to suffer from digestive issues or health issues. When researching Parkinson's disease in an effort to do all I could for my mum, I discovered that sufferers of the condition were found to be lacking in butyric acid. I quickly put my mum on a quality product containing it, and the benefits were undeniable.

Healthy bacteria play a role in almost every aspect of our health, supporting heart health, lowering cholesterol, boosting energy, balancing hormones and even preventing depression. I know! How fabulous. However, as with anything that we are putting into our bodies, it is important to take the right thing at the right time. This is why I strongly recommend a consultation with a knowledgeable health adviser who will not only be able to establish the correct blend for your needs but monitor your progress too.

Meanwhile, there are foods that encourage both pre and probiotics, such as fermented plant foods (e.g. tempeh, miso, sauerkraut, kimchi and kefir), bananas, beans, blueberries, nuts and wholegrains.

Digestive Enzymes

Whilst our own bodies produce enzymes to help break down the fats, proteins and sugars in the food we eat, we sometimes need extra support, especially as we age.

Proteases	break down proteins.
Lipases	break down fat.
Amylases	break down carbohydrates.

So strong and effective are these enzymes that they are used in many cleaning products: lipase is added to detergents; proteases remove human sweat, blood and egg; amylases remove starch residues from chocolate, gravies and pasta.

Taking digestive enzymes appropriately can help the absorption and transportation of nutrients while your own digestive enzymes are struggling, and can prevent bloating and gas.

There are a number of over-the-counter products available and most will have derivatives of natural compounds found in foods.

Here are a few examples:

- Pineapples and papayas – both contain proteases known as papain and bromelain
- Mangoes contain amylases
- Honey contains proteases and amylase together with other digestive enzymes
- Bananas contain amylases
- Avocados contain lipase
- Kefir (fermented milk) contains lipases, proteases and lactases

- **Sauerkraut (fermented cabbage) contains a variety of digestive enzymes and is also a probiotic**
- **Kimchi (fermented vegetables) has a range of digestive enzymes including proteases, lipases and amylases, and is fermented with healthy bacteria**
- **Miso (fermented soy beans) has lactases, amylases, proteases and amylases**
- **Kiwi fruit is a popular addition in digestive enzyme products as it contains actinidain, which helps digest proteins.**

One of my favourite supports for digestion is apple cider vinegar. Taking two teaspoons in a little water, 20 minutes before your meal, naturally works with your stomach acids.

As always, have a chat with your health adviser to ensure these foods are for you (e.g. unripe papayas are not suitable for pregnant women).

Chapter 4
The Perfect Poo!

Earlier, you met the digestive team, and you now know the important individual jobs that they do. When they are all working efficiently and in harmony, collectively they will help you produce a perfect poo!

The colour and consistency of poo is a good indicator of your gut health, so do take time to know what yours looks like. It matters!

Colour

Sometimes clients come to see me with what they think is a bowel issue, but I can tell from the description of their stools that the issue is more likely to be a stomach or liver problem. Old blood cells are transported out of the body via your stool, and that's what gives it its natural mid-brown colour. If you find that your stool is often a mustardy/yellow or a clay colour, that indicates some dysbiosis in your gut, or possible liver and gallbladder issues. Of course, there are certain foods, supplements and medications that will alter the colour of your stool, so bear that in mind when having a check!

Consistency

Your stool should be fully formed with no/few cracks. It should not be runny or mushy, neither should it be rock hard and bullet-like! Ideally it should have the consistency of toothpaste.

The Bristol stool scale was developed at the Bristol Royal Infirmary as a clinical assessment tool in 1997. Since that time it has become a global reference chart for health practitioners.

Bristol Stool Chart

Type 1	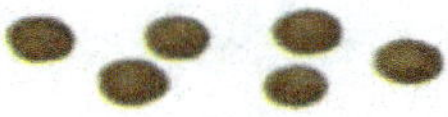	Separate hard lumps, like nuts (hard to pass)
Type 2	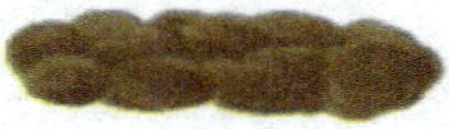	Sausage-shaped but lumpy
Type 3		Like a sausage but with cracks on the surface
Type 4	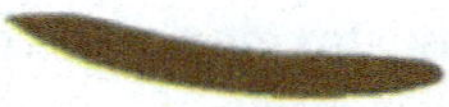	Like a sausage or snake, smooth and soft (the perfect poo!)
Type 5	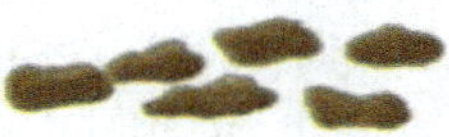	Soft blobs with clear-cut edges (passed easily)
Type 6	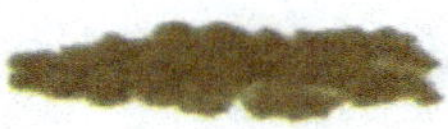	Fluffy pieceswith ragged edges, a mushy stool
Type 7	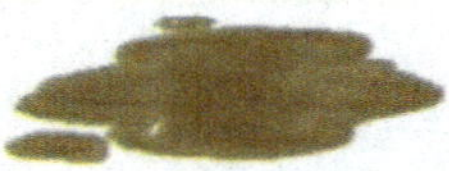	Watery, no solid pieces, entirely liquid

Important!

If you notice mucous or blood present, this could indicate a serious underlying bowel issue and I advise you to get it checked out. You can try natural solutions such as slippery elm powder, Boswelia, glutamine, etc., but it is important to know what you are dealing with. Many bowel conditions – from cancer to ulcerative colitis – present with similar symptoms.

Chapter 5

Signs of Nutrient Deficiencies

Earlier I mentioned the breakdown of our car after our friend Trevor put diesel in the tank instead of petrol. After Steve picked himself off the floor and found his voice again, he asked Trevor why he hadn't noticed his mistake before the car ground to a halt. Trevor admitted that he thought the car 'didn't feel right' but hadn't associated the change in performance with the filling up of the fuel. He said he'd noticed an increased sluggishness and decided he would stop at the next garage to have an assessment. However, as the journey continued, the performance of the car deteriorated quite dramatically – with lights coming on the dashboard, smoke billowing under the bonnet and a defiant shuddering STOP – long before a garage appeared in sight.

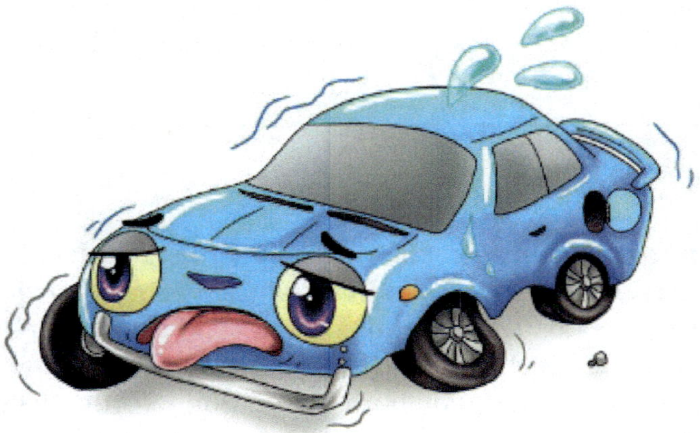

Just as a car breaking down gives us clues that it needs attention, our bodies also quickly let us know when things are not working efficiently. OK, we might not exude smoke and blow up, but some of us do shudder to a halt! If any of you have experienced chronic fatigue, you'll know what I mean. That feeling of being so utterly weak ... just awful.

I can recall a time I was in such a low state that the thought of lifting my arm to scratch the itch on my head was too overwhelming; when the effort of speaking was too demanding. Little did I know then that I had developed an intolerance to eggs, tomatoes and mushrooms – not ideal for a vegetarian! I also discovered, during my studies, that I had an issue with a group of foods known as FODMAPs (see pages 67–71). These are all perfectly healthy foods for most people but, for me, they were diesel in my petrol tank. When I think back, the signs were all there, but I wasn't paying attention, or rather I wasn't appreciating the significance.

Today, as always, the brain lets us know when our nutritional bank is running low on supplies. Take magnesium, for example. If you are lacking in this mineral, the brain gives you an early clue – and you notice it. It's that pesky old twitchy eye muscle! There, the brain has done its job. It sent out the signal and you sit with your flickering eye. Do you rush off to get some magnesium-rich food? No! You might enjoy the sensation (hey, some people do!), or ask your friends if they can see it, maybe even have a bit of a laugh about it, but increasing your magnesium intake isn't even in your thoughts. Hmmm ... so the brain has to up the ante. Ok then, how about some cramps in your legs and feet? There, that ought to do it. Nope. You run around slapping your legs (winking away) but still no magnesium. Alright, time for some serious intervention ... now you're getting headaches. In fact, the brain has decided you need a migraine as you have ignored all the other signs. Finally, you are heading to the chemist. For a magnesium supplement? No – for pain killers! Oh dear. Well, how about adding some constipation then? Surely now that you have four clear signs of magnesium deficiency you will get the message? Hooray! At last you are heading back to the chemist ... but not for magnesium, you get some laxatives. Aaaggghh!

Now it might not seem the end of the world to be spending your days winking at folk, slapping your leg and living on painkillers and laxatives but ... and it's a big but ... if you are ignoring those early signs of magnesium deficiency, you are now more vulnerable to developing conditions associated with magnesium deficiency, including heart disease. All your muscles need magnesium to function efficiently, and there is no more precious muscle than your heart. You are lacking in magnesium, and have been for some time, so the heart could be next to succumb. Or maybe you will become depressed. Magnesium helps with the balance of dopamine levels (a neurotransmitter connected with mood, anxiety and behaviour).

Tongue Tied to Health

How about that tongue of yours? Have you checked it lately? Oh, you noticed the thick white coating did you – great! What did you do about it? Ignoring it or scraping it might get rid of it, but it hasn't dealt with the crucial matter of why it was there!

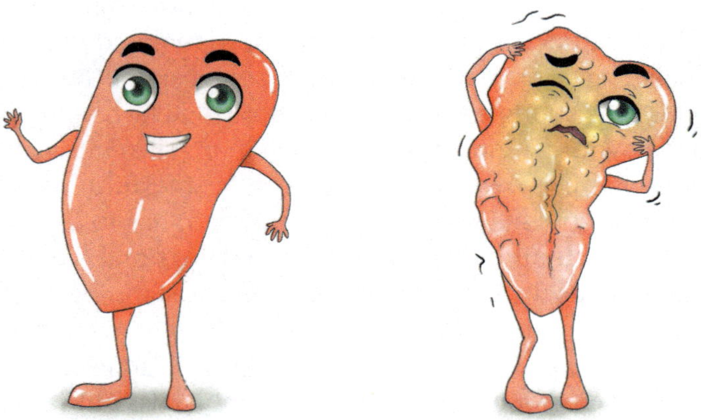

The tongue is an extension of your digestive tract and a healthy tongue should ideally look like a little kitten's tongue with no splits, cracks or coatings. At the time of writing, I have looked at over 10,000 individual tongues and they each tell a story!

In simple terms, your tongue is telling you the following:

- **Thick white coating:** This can signify a lack of healthy bacteria in your intestines. We need healthy bacteria to support our immune system, aid the absorption of nutrients and encourage regular bowel movements. Investing in a probiotic supplement or fermented food will help.

- **Thick yellow coating:** This can indicate that a food intolerance exists, especially if the coating is 'greasy' and towards the back of the tongue. Of course, what you eat and drink will affect the colour of your tongue, so before you recoil in horror at your almost brown-coloured coating, remember if you've had anything to eat or drink that would have caused the discolouration (coffee being a common culprit) and assess your tongue at different times of the day.

- **Scalloped edges:** Scalloped edges: This may mean that your spleen (that mysterious organ that no-one seems to know much about) is less than happy. That's important to know given that your spleen plays a big role in your immune system and helps manage your red and white blood cells. If you've had your tonsils and/or appendix removed, you might want to take extra special care of this hard-working but little recognised organ.

- **A central split:** Generally, this relates to your stomach acids and implies that they are weak or depleted. Apple cider vinegar (2 tsp in warm water) taken 20 minutes before meals will help to support them. You can also buy digestive enzymes in supplement form and/or increase your intake of fermented foods, such as kombucha, sauerkraut or kefir.

- **Bright red:** This can indicate a deficiency of the B vitamins, particularly vitamin B12.

- **Burning tongue:** This a sign that you may need to top up your B12, zinc and iron stores.
- **Geographic tongue:** These are lesions and patches (that look like little islands) but which are generally symptomless.

Prevention is Better Than Cure

Apart from our tongue, our body also gives us many other clues that nutritional support is needed.

There's the old saying that prevention is better than cure, and we could prevent many health conditions arising if we just stopped and took note of the signs and signals our bodies are giving us. Sadly, if we DO take notice, we often treat the symptom rather than the cause.

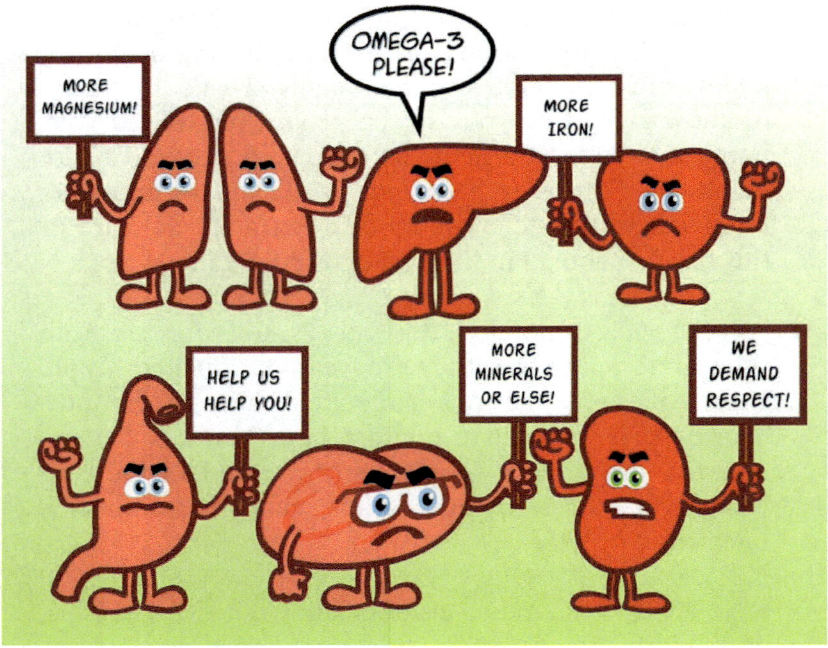

Illustration by Jeremy Woods.

Here are some signs of common nutrient deficiencies:

- **Vitamin B12 (cobalamin):** low energy, pins and needles, numbness, swollen tongue, lack of balance
- **Vitamin B2 (riboflavin):** migraines, pale skin, sensitivity to light, sore tongue and lips
- **Calcium:** muscle aches, insomnia, tooth decay, brittle nails, poor growth
- **Vitamin C:** dry wrinkly skin, splitting hair, poor immune system, painful joints
- **Vitamin D:** migraines, aching bones, sweaty head
- **Iron:** fatigue, impaired cognitive function, hair loss, restless legs
- **Magnesium:** twitchy eye muscles, cramps, headaches, constipation, low moods
- **Zinc:** acne, boils, gum disease, forgetfulness.

Later, I will list the top foods containing these and other key nutrients.

Chapter 6
Food Intolerances

If you can't explain why you're not feeling 100% when your diet and exercise regime look to be fine, you may have a food intolerance.

A food intolerance is not the same as a food allergy. Just as it has always done, the body needs to let us know when we are being invaded or attacked. With an allergic response, the body releases chemicals (such as histamine) that trigger an immediate symptom. You might feel a tingling sensation on your lips or tongue, or you might notice welts appearing. In the worst-case scenario, your oesophagus would close and you'd suffer an anaphylactic shock. So, people with allergies usually know they have them!

Intolerances are different. When you eat a food that you are intolerant to, your immune system perceives specific food molecules as 'invaders'. This affects the autonomic nervous system (our inbuilt 'fight or flight' response) and for a split second we are on full alert. At this precise time, our muscles 'fail', we produce adrenalin and we also produce antibodies if the invader is entering our system. All of this takes place without us noticing! Yet the impact is immense.

In your small intestine, you have trillions of villi, little finger-like protrusions that help distribute the nutrients to your cells. When you are intolerant to a food and experience the 'fight or flight' response, all your muscles fail, and so do the villi. They immediately lay flat. When that happens, all your nutrients pass through your system without ever reaching the cells they were destined to feed. Once the danger has passed, the villi stand upright again[1] – and you haven't noticed a thing.

The first symptom you may feel is hunger; you've had a hearty breakfast at 7.30 am but by 9.00 am you are ravenous. That's because you didn't absorb the nutrients from your breakfast. You might also notice tiredness – it's one of those days you are struggling through, yawning, unable to concentrate and feeling generally blah. Hunger and tiredness are common symptoms of food intolerances but not always investigated. Perhaps the symptom that may get your attention is digestive discomfort. You may experience anything from bloating and gas, reflux and heartburn to irregular bowel movements caused by inflammation and damage to your intestinal tract. Before rushing off for Gaviscon, omeprazole or Wind-Eze, consider having a food intolerance test.

Over time, if you continue to eat food(s) you are not tolerating, the impact will lead to nutritional deficiencies. It is these deficiencies that cause the symptoms and they will be different for each individual. Many common ailments such as migraines, eczema, joint pain, digestive issues, fatigue and even depression often have a food culprit at their source.

Food Intolerance Testing

There are various methods of testing for food intolerances, including blood tests, PST (percutaneous skin testing), hair analysis and muscle testing (applied kinesiology).

When I first heard about muscle testing I was very sceptical. I Googled it (as you do!) and concluded that it was a load of old twaddle. When it was included in one of the courses I

1. Unless you have coeliac disease (an extreme intolerance to gluten). In this case, the villi become 'sticky' with the gluten and are not able to stand upright.

was studying I was less than impressed but went along with it because it was part of the course and I wasn't studying in order to set up a practice (ha!) or go preaching to the world (double ha!) I was studying because I was so very unwell and the only advice I had been given was to "take this medication for the rest of your life".

During my studies, muscle testing revealed that I was intolerant to eggs, tomatoes and mushrooms. The test required that I eliminate them from my diet. I did so ... and I could not believe the impact! Almost immediately my intense fatigue lifted, and my digestive system improved dramatically. Could it be that simple? Yes, it could. From that time on I have never needed any medication to manage my symptoms of ulcerative colitis and have been in complete remission. As time went by, I re-introduced all of them and can now enjoy a lovely vegetarian breakfast featuring all three. However, if I am feeling rundown or that something is 'not quite right' in my body, then I eliminate them until I feel my system is more settled.

I cannot begin to tell you how excited I was by this – very simple – revelation! I wanted to shout it from the rooftops. Why weren't we taking intolerances more seriously? Sure, I had been tested for coeliac disease (extreme intolerance to gluten) as part of the many tests I had whilst they were trying to figure out why I was so unwell. (For many years, my doctor had dismissed all my symptoms as a 'combination of perimenopause and IBS', and I had believed him until I was completely debilitated, even though it was evident that not all pre-menopausal women were in a constant state of collapse!) I didn't have an issue with gluten, nor indeed with dairy. Nope. I had issues with the very healthy organic eggs, home-grown tomatoes and mushrooms that made up a large part of my vegetarian diet.

When I decided to go into practice, I made sure that food intolerance tests were an integral part of the consultations. I combined my conventional knowledge with my holistic knowledge and designed and developed a quick and effective muscle testing method. It's great for the needle-averse! I also encouraged the students I was mentoring to include it in their studies too. Very often, it's barely given a second thought, especially in conventional nutrition where gluten and dairy take the spotlight. I appreciated that not everyone would be comfortable with muscle testing, so I also offered (and still do offer) a range of testing methods including blood samples and hair mineral analysis – anything that will enable me to help find the food friends and foes for my clients.

Case Study

Sandra was an exceptionally fit and healthy 64-year-old. A high-performing athlete for most of her life, she was still competing in challenging triathlons and marathons and her performance could knock spots off those half her age. Her usual regime included 100k bike rides three times a week, 15k runs every day and regular swimming sessions. She also did weight training. All of these exercises would be increased in the lead up to her events. Her diet (on paper at least) was exemplary. She had paid for a dietician to work out what was best for her before, during and after exercise and was following it religiously. Yet Sandra was overweight and miserable.

She went to her doctor to ask why she wasn't losing weight, and he simply told her to "eat less and move more". (Really?!) She was understandably devastated. A friend of hers had been to see me and suggested she should come along. Reluctantly she did. Her whole demeanour reflected the frustration and hopelessness that she was experiencing.

Through her sighs, she answered my questions. I was beginning to pick up signs that she had quite acute nutritional deficiencies despite her healthy diet. One look at her tongue confirmed my suspicion that she had food intolerances and had likely had them for a while. "But I never have gluten or dairy and I'm following a clean-eating diet" she sighed. Great. "But some of the foods you are eating are clearly not your friends", I told her. She agreed to a food intolerance test and it revealed that she was hugely intolerant to spinach, kale, broccoli, almonds, blueberries and coconut. Most of which went into her 'healthy' smoothie every morning!

The turnaround in her health was (as I knew it would be) dramatic. She not only felt better, had more focus and concentration (which she hadn't realised was a problem until she got it back) but she also lost weight.

Case Study

I also recall the story of Jessica, an ex-nurse who had been suffering from malaise and migraines for 17 years. With no obvious reason for her symptoms, her doctors had put her on strong painkillers and antidepressants. On a good day, Jessica could struggle down the path to her mailbox. On a bad day, she was bedridden in a darkened room. She had far more bad days than good.

Again, it was a friend who suggested that Jessica come along for a consultation with me. Like Sandra, Jessica was intolerant to 'healthy' food, with her biggest culprit being bananas. I saw her on a Monday and she had the muscle test, so the results were instant. She asked how soon she might expect to feel better. I told her that everyone was different, of course, but now that we had identified some clear food enemies, she should be hopeful that it wouldn't be too long. She called me on Friday of the same week exclaiming, "Don't tell me it was that simple?!'"After 17 years of what she described as a 'living hell' she was back on the right path ***in just a week****, after just one hour's consultation with me. (Gosh, I love this job!)*

Well, Jessica was on a mission after that! She went to her doctor, her specialist, the newspaper, the national radio station, the District Health Board, even the Minister for Health at the time. She was outraged that not one person had considered food intolerance tests throughout her years of misery and felt she had been 'fobbed off' with medication.

As you can imagine, I have no end of similar stories (another book beckons!) but I will end with just one more. This one touches my heart every time I relay it because it had such a profound effect not only on the little girl I was treating, but all her lovely family.

Case Study

Little Kate was 5 years old. I had given a presentation to her dad's place of work and he approached me afterwards to ask if I could help his little girl. Her hair was falling out and no-one could understand why. The usual tests had been done and a counsellor had been brought in just in case it was stress related. No joy. I agreed to see beautiful little Kate, and her mum and dad joined her at the first appointment.

It was immediately apparent that Kate also had a skin problem. "Oh, we are seeing a dermatologist for that," said her mum. As I proceeded with the consultation, it was also evident that Kate had awful digestive problems. She had been constipated almost from birth. "But we are seeing a gastroenterologist for that." Hmmm... I then did some food intolerance testing and picked up that Kate was intolerant to gluten, soy, eggs and borderline intolerant to dairy. I assured her mum that as soon as we eliminated these foods from her diet, the digestive system would work, and once that was doing what it should, her cells would receive the nutrients they needed, her skin would clear up and her hair would grow back. Kate's mum was delighted, although I could see she was still a little bit cautious about being too excited (after 5 years of tests and appointments, all to no avail, who could blame her).

Just 4 weeks later, little Kate came back for her review and it was an absolute joy to see her looking so different.

As predicted, her digestive system was working well, her new foods were suiting her system, her skin had cleared and there was wonderful evidence of new hair growth. That would be fantastic enough if that were the end of the story but there's more and, for me, it is the most wonderful part. Kate's mum had tears in her eyes as she said, "We have a new child. We have never known her so happy and engaged with everything she does. We have other children and had concluded that Kate was the quiet one. She would do puzzles or colouring in, read books, etc., but never seemed to want to take part in anything demanding or exciting. She was happy enough in herself – or so we thought. Since the change in diet, she dances, plays, laughs – she is HAPPY!"

That's because 90% of serotonin (our 'feel-good' brain chemical) is manufactured in the gut, and little Kate's gut had not been working since she'd been born.

I saw Kate's mum some months later and she told me that Kate had reached the top of her class. That's so good to hear, given that prior to the change in her diet her teachers had said she was struggling and didn't seem to be able to concentrate.

Now, Kate's mum wasn't setting out to harm her child, Sandra wasn't intentionally tripping herself up with her choice of smoothie, and Jessica most certainly didn't realise that her organic food choices were keeping her practically bed-ridden for 17 years. That's the impact that food intolerances can have. I urge you, if you or your loved ones are experiencing an ongoing health issue, skin issue, weight issue or even depression, please do consider having a food intolerance test. And be aware, that it's not always gluten at fault here! So many specialists test for gluten and that's as far as the tests go, but as you've seen, it can be any food!

If you're not ready to commit to a test, try keeping a food and symptom diary. Recording what you eat and drink in one column with symptoms in another can highlight potential culprits. Remember, intolerances generate delayed symptoms, so be aware that your 10 am banana could be responsible for your 3 pm headache.

Foods to Look Out For

It's worth knowing that six foods are responsible for 80% of intolerances:

Food	Where you might find it
Yeast	Mainly found in bread, alcohol, marmite/vegemite, and most processed food. So, if you are using packets and jars frequently, check the label
Dairy products	Butter, cream, cheese, ice cream, yoghurt
Gluten	Products containing wheat, spelt, barley, rye and oats; biscuits, cereals, pasta
Tomatoes	Pasta sauce, baked bean sauce, ketchup
Eggs	Biscuits, scones, cakes, mayonnaise
Soy products and anything containing lecithin (food additive 322)	Tofu, miso

Sometimes, you may only have a sensitivity to a food. Whilst this wouldn't warrant elimination of it from your diet, you'd need to be careful that you don't each too much of it in any one day, and be mindful not to have it with any other foods to which you are sensitive. This is because their cumulative effect would mimic an intolerance.

Sensitivities can sometimes progress into intolerances, so keep an eye on any suspects and have them re-tested from time to time.

Gluten

Gluten is a protein by-product of wheat, barley, rye and some oats. It is a sticky protein and can cause digestive issues, not because you cannot tolerate it, but because your engine is not robust enough to break it down.

Gluten is known to aggravate eczema and dry skin conditions, so you may notice a difference in any dry skin patches when you eliminate it from your diet.

Mood and behavioural conditions including anxiety, depression, ADHD and Asperger's have been shown to improve when a gluten-free diet is followed.

Lactose

Lactose is a type of sugar found in milk and milk products. Being lactose intolerant means you are unable to properly digest lactose owing to a deficiency of an enzyme in your small intestine called lactase. As a result, the milk sugars can't be broken down into simpler forms that can be absorbed into your bloodstream.

Some products listed as non-dairy, such as powdered coffee creamer and whipped toppings, may contain lactose if they contain ingredients that are derived from milk. When you read food labels, look for words such as casein, whey, curds, milk by-products, dry milk solids and non-fat dry milk powder, and watch for food additive numbers 325–329 and 966. If any of these ingredients are on the label, the product probably contains lactose.

A lactose intolerance interferes with the absorption of tryptophan in the intestines, and therefore reduces tryptophan levels in your blood, and this can result in low moods.

The processing of yoghurt makes lactose more tolerable, so it's possible that you can have that without any ill effects. I suggest you try eating a few spoonfuls of yoghurt and monitor how you feel afterwards.

Chapter 7

The Microbiome and Our Gut–Brain Axis

I couldn't move on to the next part of the book without acknowledging our gut–brain axis. As mentioned earlier, the biochemical signals between our gastrointestinal tract and our central nervous system influence everything from our weight to our mood and from our bowel movements to our sleep patterns. These communication signals work through our vagus nerve, which runs between our brain and our gut and is referred to as the gut–brain axis.

Known as our second brain, the microbiota in our gut play an important role in every aspect of our health. I remember being particularly intrigued by the work of the gastroenterologist Dr. Stephen Collins, who had been studying the impact of antibiotics on mood and behaviour. Having seen a clear link, his research led him to look at the impact of probiotics and how they affected conditions like depression and insomnia. I don't condone animal experiments at all, but his work led him to experiment with faecal transplants, showing that introducing new strains of bacteria from a calm and happy mouse to an aggressive mouse caused the aggressive mouse to become calm. He was one of the pioneers proving the direct link between microbiota and mood. Fast forward, and faecal microbiota transplant (FMT)[2] is now widely used in humans and has been very effective in

2. Fecal microbiota transplantation (FMT) was first described in China in the 4th century by Ge Hong.

the control of conditions such as autism and other behavioural disorders.

FMT is also used to help those with chronic bowel conditions. Our ancestors used to eat roots, shoots, leaves, fruit and berries, all with remnants of soil on them. This would feed the healthy bacteria in their gut and strengthen their immune systems. Not only did they eat soil, they would sleep on it and bathed with it. When the Tyrolean Iceman was discovered, scientists revealed he had a vastly different range and spread of healthy bacteria to those in humans today. Indeed, many of our modern bowel conditions such as ulcerative colitis can develop due to the fact that we don't have the right bacteria in our gut from soils. Soil-based probiotics have been introduced and have been proven to be very effective.

Eating fermented foods is also very beneficial for encouraging the growth of healthy bacteria in the gut, so spread some sauerkraut on your crackers! Or, do as I do, and make your own yoghurt. You can create your own super-blend by choosing the species of healthy bacteria you want to focus on (see pages 28–29) and keep your health and your gut in tip top condition.

Part 2

Natural Remedies for Common Health Issues

Whilst there are hundreds of illnesses and diseases ranging from mild to severe, I have focused on the most common that I see in my clinics. I emphasise again that we are all different. The advice here is generic and there may be reasons why you can't follow some of the suggestions.

Choosing fresh, seasonal produce (ideally growing your own where possible) and eating a good range of all foods will provide your body with the nutrients it needs to keep you healthy (except for food intolerances of course). Using food as medicine is as old as man himself; *"Let food be thy medicine and medicine be thy food"* Hippocrates said in 400 BC. Today is no exception. All fruits and vegetables have healing properties and, when eaten with knowledge, you can prevent many health issues arising, or reverse those that have arisen.

Chapter 1
Digestive Disorders

When we experience any digestive discomfort, we must take note and address the symptom as soon as possible. (Got to keep our engine firing on all cylinders!) This doesn't mean resorting to prescribed medications all the time. I am so frustrated at the amount of people – including babies – who are given all sorts of medications to treat a symptom rather than investigations to address the cause.

Case Study

Take Stan for instance. Lovely 84-year-old Stan who, in the words of his son, was "projectile vomiting like a baby" every time he ate. Stan had been seen by a raft of doctors and specialists, had been subjected to all manner of tests, including a gastroscopy and an MRI scan, and was taking several medications, including one for nausea (despite that fact that he said he never felt nausea!)

The medics were scratching their heads with no idea why Stan was having such issues, as the tests had revealed that he was functioning perfectly well. They were at a loss and couldn't help him. Their only solution was to give him all the medication they could think of ... and he still had severe reflux.

Stan's son had attended one of my health awareness presentations and spoke to me afterwards. He said that food intolerances had not been considered and was hopeful that this could be the answer for his Dad. I agreed to do a home visit to Stan and took my food intolerance test kit with me. However, on entering Stan's tiny apartment, it struck me that there was no dining table, no designated area to eat in fact. I asked him where he ate his meals. He pulled out a very low coffee table from under a larger table (that housed all his medication, some books, photos and a sweet little pot plant). "I use this", he said, as he bent almost in half over it. That was it! That was the answer.

The digestive tract is simply one long tube from oesophagus to bowel – and Stan was kinking his tube. He had never needed scans and probes and medication, he simply needed to sit up straight! After my visit, his son made him a special tray that was fitted to his chair. It could be folded out of the way and swivelled round at meal times. I asked for it to be made at a height that meant Stan had to sit as upright as he could – and he never experienced reflux again (and didn't need any more medication). If only someone had taken the time to investigate the cause of Stan's ongoing reflux rather than treat the symptom, he'd have been spared a long and upsetting round of unnecessary, resource-intensive tests and procedures.

The following are amongst the most common digestive issues that my clients come to see me about.

Reflux

Think of a cauldron full of acid; acid so strong it would burn a hole through your dining room table. Well, that's what you have inside you, albeit not in a cauldron! Your stomach (gastric) acids are so powerful that they could even melt metal. Little wonder then that when things are not working efficiently in your stomach you can experience an intense burning sensation. To understand why and, more to the point, prevent it occurring, here's an overview of what's taking place inside.

There is a sphincter that opens and shuts when food passes from your oesophagus to your stomach. You have a mucosal lining along your intestinal tract from which mucous is 'collected' naturally and mixed with your food. The mucous forms a layer on the lining and is one way the stomach and upper small intestine protect themselves against the otherwise damaging effects of stomach acid. This mucosal lining helps to 'stick' the sphincter closed once it shuts. If this process isn't working well, stomach acids can escape into your oesophagus, causing painful burning and reflux. It is being caused by an erosion of the mucosal lining.

There are some usual suspects that contribute to reflux, including spicy foods. Chocolate can also be a cause for some people. Researchers discovered that the high levels of serotonin (a neurotransmitter that helps regulate mood, emotions, appetite and sleep) found in chocolate can relax the lower oesophageal sphincter, allowing stomach acids to enter. If you are not sure if chocolate affects you in this way, try eating a small portion (four or five squares) and see how you feel within an hour.

Of course, it makes sense to prevent the stomach acids from bubbling away in the first place and you can do this by following some of the digestive tips on pages 22–26 and trying some of the natural supports below.

Natural supports include:

- Food combining (eating fruit first, followed by vegetables, then carbohydrates and finally protein – meat or fish) will mean that your stomach acids are only dealing with one food group at a time and it will help stop them bubbling
- 2 teaspoons of apple cider vinegar in a small glass of room-temperature water taken 20 minutes before eating
- 1 teaspoon of slippery elm powder in a little water – any time of the day. This will help repair the mucosal lining and reduce inflammation

- Have some raw food (e.g. a piece of fruit, a carrot, some salad) 20 minutes before your main meal to help stimulate your digestive enzymes
- A teaspoon of baking soda in room-temperature water (helps put out the fire!)

Indigestion

I've found that clients' descriptions for indigestion (also known as dyspepsia) varies from 'uncomfortable tummy ache' to 'extreme pain' experienced in the upper part of their abdomen after eating, with frequency ranging from 'every so often' to 'daily'. Food and symptom diaries are very helpful to establish exactly what is happening and when, and, if indeed, it's something other than indigestion.

Natural supports include:

- Being mindful of food combinations (the more confusion on your plate, the harder your digestive organs will need to work) – see the tip above for reflux
- Sitting up straight and chewing thoroughly
- Eating smaller portions
- Peppermint tea
- Ginger tea

Gallstones

If you are aged 50 or over, the chances are that you've got some 'sludge' in your gallbladder, and quite possibly a few gallstones rattling around in there as well. Most often, they won't cause you any harm and you won't even be aware that they are there. They can break up, dissolve and pass through your system naturally without you noticing a thing. It's only when they become large or numerous that they might become troublesome. In extreme cases, they can be very painful and even life-threatening.

If you believe (or know) you have gallstones, get to know which type you have, their size and their location. It really helps put you in control in order to know how best to tackle them. If you opt for surgery, that's fine, but surgery isn't always necessary. I have seen far too many people who have had their gallbladders taken out needlessly, and who are then left coping with a new digestive issue on their hands.

As this book is all about raising awareness, here are some typical Q&As on gallstones.

Q: What are gallstones?

A: Gallstones are the formation of crystalline deposits in the gallbladder.

Q: What causes them?

A: They usually form when bile liquid hardens. The most common reason for this is due to a diet containing too much protein (Atkins followers beware!), but skipping meals also heightens your risk. When you eat, the gallbladder contracts and squeezes bile through a little duct to help emulsify fats and oils in your food. If you regularly leave longer than 3 hours a day between meals, this may lead to a sludgy, if not stony, gallbladder. Some studies have also linked food intolerances to gallstone formation, with common foods such as eggs, poultry, pork, corn, beans and nuts high on the list.

Q: What are the symptoms?

A: Most commonly there is nausea (especially after eating a fatty meal) and vomiting. A severe attack is accompanied by intense pain in the right side of the abdomen and sometimes in the shoulder blade area.

Q: How can I prevent them?

A: The number one rule is to eat regularly! Going longer than 3 hours will cause the bile fluid to solidify and weaken the function of the gallbladder – just as any muscle becomes weak when not used regularly. You should also avoid high fat foods.

Natural supports include:

- Drinking warm water with lemon juice or apple cider vinegar to help dissolve any stones that may be forming
- Olive oil and lemon juice together to support the health of your gallbladder and naturally flush away small deposits
- Soy lecithin to assist in the emulsification of fats and oils in your diet, reducing your risk of gallstones
- Herbs such as milk thistle, peppermint and golden seal also have proven benefits.

Gall bladder removal

When I opened my first clinic in New Zealand, I was utterly staggered by the amount of people I was seeing who had had their gallbladders removed. More staggering, and upsetting, was the fact that most of these clients told me that they had received no dietary advice before, during or after surgery. I was shocked to think this was so, so I set off to the hospital to speak with the dietician there.

Apart from jumping out of her seat because someone had actually discovered her very remotely located office, the dietician looked surprised that I had come to ask about the advice being given to gallstone patients. She disappeared into a cupboard and came back dusting off a very poorly photocopied one-sided A4 piece of paper and dangled it proudly in front of me. "There's this – if they want it" she announced. I gazed at the faded words and asked when she had last given this 'advice' sheet out. She simply shrugged and couldn't recall. It had been a while, she admitted, because "no-one has asked for it'" Sigh. I offered to prepare a (readable) fact sheet, but the offer was declined because I was running a private practice. Fair enough. How about I prepare it anyway, no logo, no name, and she could present it to the District Health Board for approval? No, that wouldn't be a good idea. Hmmm. So, what did she think we needed to do to resolve the situation and help educate people so that they were fully aware at all stages – before, during and after surgery – of their choices? She felt the existing fact sheet was good enough, it was being used all over the country, it would be "too hard" to change it anyway and she wasn't convinced that anyone would be interested in anything new as they weren't even reading what had already been produced. Aaaghh! Because they didn't know it existed!

I wasn't content to leave things at that, so I went to the local press. Not to point fingers or blame anyone (I didn't mention my experience at the hospital), merely to raise awareness that whilst surgery was one choice there were other options to consider. The article proved incredibly successful, and I was inundated with queries from people who had either already had their gallbladders removed or who were waiting for surgery. Following my prompt, one lady asked her surgeon for more information on the size and number of stones ahead of her upcoming operation. He discussed her scan results with her, and she was very surprised to see there were hardly any stones present. She decided to postpone the operation whilst she tried the natural remedies I'd recommended. Just three months later, she returned for another scan, and the stones had completely gone.

Gallstones can be life-threatening if they grow large enough to block the bile duct, so I'm definitely not suggesting that surgery should be discounted. It can, and does, save lives. However, I'm convinced that many surgeries are not warranted, so I recommend you ask for as much information as possible regarding the type, size and quantity of your stones before making any decisions.

Of course, you can certainly live without your gallbladder, but there is a consequence to its removal. Bile is still being produced, but instead of being held in your gallbladder it is now being redirected to your small intestine. If you have no issue with soy, try two teaspoons of soy lecithin granules every day (lovely in porridge oats) to help emulsify fats and oils in the absence of your gallbladder.

Just an interesting little fact to end on: the heaviest gallstone ever removed came from an 80-year-old English woman and weighed just under 6kg. Yikes!

Irritable Bowel Syndrome

Aaaghh! If there's one medical terminology for a condition that makes me angry, it's this one. Irritable Bowel Syndrome (IBS) is used as a common explanation for irregular bowel movements and/or digestive pain. Ok, so it's irritable ... but why?

I was told for years that I had IBS and I believed that I did. Why would I question my doctor? He had run a few tests that were 'all fine' (I discovered years later that they were anything but), suggested my symptoms were a combination of perimenopause and IBS, stuffed me with medication and that was that. Except it wasn't. My poor body was in complete disarray and the medication, although temporarily relieving the ever-debilitating symptoms, was only adding to the turmoil. It was only when my symptoms literally ground me to a halt on holiday in New Zealand that I discovered I had an inflammatory bowel condition called ulcerative colitis, which unfortunately had been allowed to take more of a hold than it should have because I had been incorrectly treating the symptoms as IBS.

Whenever I see clients in my clinics who present with any similar ongoing symptoms or who have assumed they have (or been diagnosed with) IBS, I always encourage a colonoscopy. This procedure uses a camera to look inside you to determine the health of your intestines. It can reveal conditions such as coeliac disease, Crohn's disease, diverticulitis and, of course, ulcerative colitis.

Here are a few of the most common symptoms associated with IBS:

- **Bloating**
- **Excess gas**
- **Lower abdominal pain**
- **A 'dragging' sensation**
- **Irregular bowel movements**
- **Mucousy stools**
- **A feeling of not emptying**

Hmmm ... so quite a few then! And each and every one of those symptoms has other potential causes, so accepting a diagnosis of IBS is not good enough, in my opinion. Not until you have thoroughly investigated and eliminated all of those other causes. In my clinical experience, I don't recall anyone ever leaving with 'IBS' after we have finally unraveled their digestive history, food choices, intolerances and eating habits.

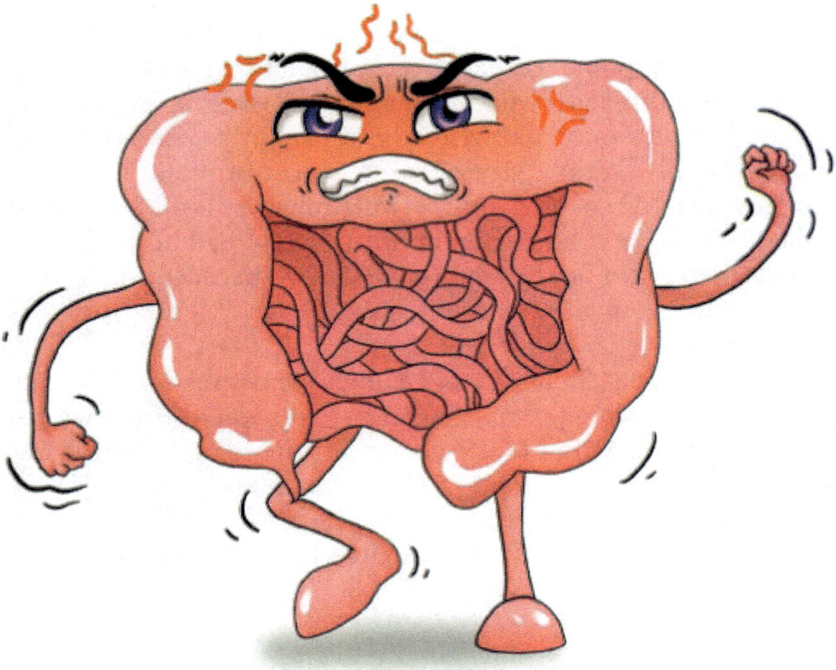

Natural supports include:

- Drinking plenty of water
- Reducing inflammation with a fish oil supplement containing at least 600 mg of EPA (look at the back of the label on your product)
- A glutamine supplement
- A probiotic
- Eating/drinking fermented foods.

Bloating/gas

There are many potential causes for this condition, including not chewing your food properly. Indeed, for those who have bad teeth, or few teeth, many digestive issues can develop at this point. Large pieces of unchewed foods, hard gristly meat, nuts, skins of fruit, etc. are meant to be pulped by your tongue, teeth and saliva. As noted earlier, there are no cutting tools inside you! If you have a very windy baby, check they have no tongue-tie. I've had quite a few cases where this was the case, and a simple release fixed all the digestive issues.

Although we have become used to having a glass of water on the table with our meals, or sipping a glass of wine, we are not really designed to have liquid and solids at the same time. We have adapted, of course and many of us don't experience any discomfort. However, if you are noticing bloating and gas, especially if you're aged over 50 years old, then try avoiding drinking when you eat. (Research advises that we should

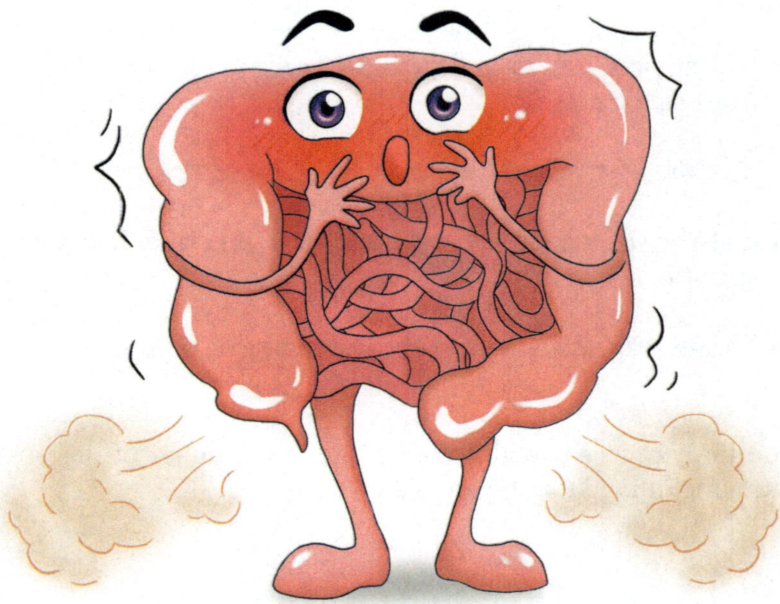

stop drinking 20 minutes before you eat and wait 40 minutes afterwards. I don't feel we need to be quite that strict and many of my clients have noticed significant improvement by simply avoiding drinks with their meals without timing the before and after.)

Sitting up straight is so important. If you are ageing, your muscles can become slacker, including the muscles that work your digestive tract. It's one of the most common reasons for digestive issues (remember poor old Stan!), and with more and more of us sitting with trays on our laps rather than up at a table, bloating is becoming more of an issue.

Our stomach acids begin to deplete as we age too and, where we may have been able to enjoy spicier food and various food combinations when we were younger, depleted stomach acids can soon change the way we eat and also the way in which we eat them.

If your bloating or gas is severe, try eating in this order:

- Fruit first or at least an hour after a meal. Avoid putting fruit with other foods, particularly grain
- Vegetables – they transit quite quickly through the digestive system
- Carbohydrates (e.g. potatoes, pasta, rice) – they take 2 hours from mouth to bowel
- Proteins (meat, fish) – they take 4 hours from mouth to bowel.

Food intolerances can also contribute to a number of digestive issues, including bloating and gas.

There are foods that naturally create gas as they are being digested and, for some systems they can be too challenging. FODMAPs is an acronym for Fermentable Oligosaccharides, Disaccharides, Monosaccharides and Polyols. These are complex names for a collection of molecules found in mostly in carbohydrate-based foods that can be poorly absorbed by some people. These carbohydrates can end up fermenting in the intestines, leading to signs of irritable bowel syndrome (IBS) or small intestinal bacterial overgrowth (SIBO).

High FODMAPs – Fruits	Low FODMAPs – Fruits
Apples	Bananas
Apricots	Blueberries
Avocado	Boysenberries
Cherries	Cantaloupe melon
Mangoes	Cranberries
Nectarines	Grapefruit
Peaches	Grapes
Pears	Honeydew melon
Plums and prunes	Kiwi fruit
Watermelon	Lemons
High concentration of fructose from canned fruit, dried fruit or fruit juice	Limes

High FODMAPs – Fruits	Low FODMAPs – Fruits
	Mandarins
	Oranges
	Passionfruit
	Raspberries
	Rhubarb
	Strawberries
	Tangelos

High FODMAPs – Vegetables	Low FODMAPs – Vegetables
Artichokes	Alfalfa shoots
Asparagus	Bamboo shoots
Beetroot	Bok choy/Pak choy
Broccoli	Carrots
Brussel sprouts	Celery
Cabbage	Corn
Cauliflower	Aubergines/Eggplant
Garlic (with large consumption)	Ginger
Fennel	Green beans
Leeks	Kumara/Sweet potato

High FODMAPs – Vegetables	Low FODMAPs – Vegetables
Mushrooms	Lettuce
Okra	Olives
Onions	Parsnips
Peas	Silverbeet/Chard
Radicchio lettuce	Spinach
Shallots	Swede
Sugar snap peas	Tomatoes
Snow peas	Turnip

High FODMAPs – Grains Level of FODMAPs is increased when these foods are eaten in large amounts:	Low FODMAPs – Grains
Rye	Amaranth
Wheat	Arrowroot
	Buckwheat
	Millet
	Spelt

High FODMAPs – Other	Low FODMAPs – Other
Lactose-Containing Foods (most dairy products)	Artificial sweeteners that do not end in -ol
	Gelato
	Glucose
	Lactose alternatives
	Lactose-free products
	Maple syrup
	Rice milk
	Sorbet
	Sugar (sucrose)
	Sweeteners

Not all foods have been tested, so the list is not complete, and not all people will react to all FODMAP categories. My advice is to place a tick beside any 'high' FODMAP food that you feel has caused discomfort. You'll soon be able to identify those that are working against you.

A word here about fermented foods: sauerkraut, for instance, uses cabbage as a base – a high FODMAP food. Many people who are following a low FODMAP diet naturally shy away from sauerkraut because of the FODMAP association. However, the fermentation process generally renders the cabbage more digestible. In fact, researchers who first developed the low FODMAP diet, and monitored its impact, discovered that a perpetual low FODMAP diet restricts food that feed healthy bacteria in the gut. They concluded that, without adding in probiotic-rich foods like sauerkraut and kefir, the inner ecosystem may be compromised. For this reason, I don't encourage clients to keep strictly to a low FODMAP diet. As mentioned, they will not *all* be your enemy. After an elimination period, try to re-introduce those that you have been excluding and note your body's response.

Natural supports include:

- **Identifying any high FODMAP foods that your system struggles with**
- **Trying a charcoal supplement to disperse gas (but do not rely on this long-term)**
- **For babies, check there is no tongue or lip-tie.**

Constipation

This is an interesting one. The definition of constipation is 'a condition in which there is difficulty in emptying the bowels, usually associated with hardened stools', and clinically it's acknowledged as passing less than three stools a week. But you can still experience constipation even if you are opening your bowels every day. Whilst small, hard stools are perhaps the most widely recognised evidence of constipation, you can be constipated even if you have loose runny stools most often associated with diarrhoea.

As we've already seen, there is teamwork involved in the production of a stool and, often, it's nothing to do with the bowel at all – it can be down to the inefficiency of the other digestive organs. That's why it's important to take notice of the colour and consistency of your stool as it gives a clue as to which organ may be contributing to the constipation. "Oh dear, I don't ever look" is a fairly common response when I ask about stool size and colour. Well look! It's a perfectly natural bodily function that every single human being performs all their life.

If you have any kind of digestive discomfort, especially erratic bowel movements, get to understand more about what the cause could be.

Natural supports include:

- Drinking plenty of water throughout the day
- Increasing the fibre and roughage in your diet
- Taking a magnesium supplement
- Adding psyllium husks to a smoothie
- Taking slippery elm powder (1 tsp in a little warm water).

Diarrhoea

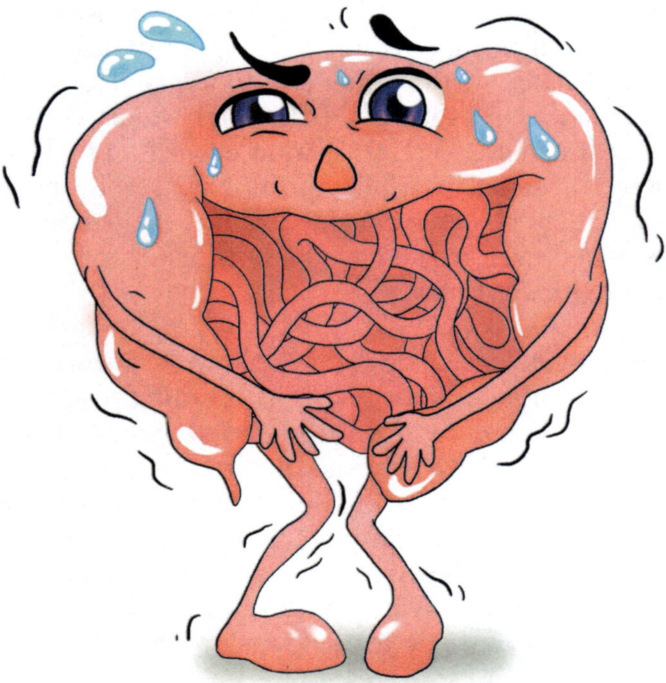

You know the feeling ... all of a sudden you need to 'go'! (And there's never a handy toilet, is there?) Diarrhoea is not pleasant at all. It is usually associated with an urgency to empty your bowels, accompanied by very loose watery stools and stomach cramps. Fortunately, it doesn't (or shouldn't) last long and we're back to normal within 24–36 hours.

However, if you are experiencing ongoing urgent, loose bowel movements then it's crucial to establish the cause.

Most commonly, triggers would include:

- Contaminated food – either something that was not properly cooked or that wasn't handled or stored correctly
- Overuse of vitamin C supplements
- Parasites
- Side effects of certain medications (metformin, for diabetes, is a common culprit)
- Overuse of magnesium supplements
- Food intolerances

Natural supports include:

- 1 tsp slippery elm powder in a little warm water
- Ginger
- Blueberries
- Chamomile tea.

It's important to stay hydrated too, so sip on cool, previously boiled, water. You can add an electrolyte powder mix to it if you are feeling particularly weak, to help replenish valuable nutrients. Meanwhile, avoid caffeine and gluten.

Diverticular Disease

Diverticula are small pouches that form on the walls of the intestines. Diverticulosis arises when there are multiple diverticula and quite often causes no immediate symptoms. Diverticulitis is caused by an infection in the small pouches/ diverticula causing chronic swelling, inflammation and pain, and mostly affects older people.

Whilst a high fibre diet helps prevent attacks, when you are having a flare up you should reduce the amount of fibre residue you intake to less than 10 grams a day. This will decrease bowel volume so that the infection can heal. To achieve this, you should avoid whole grains and opt for refined white bread, bagels, buns, etc., and plain cereals such as flakes as opposed to muesli (intolerances permitting). Avoid nuts and seeds but eat soft fruit like peaches, melons, bananas, etc. Unpulped fruit juice is OK. Finally, avoid vegetables from the cruciferous family such as broccoli, cauliflower, Brussel sprouts, cabbage, kale, Swiss chard, etc. As the attack wears off, gradually re-introduce fibre back into your diet and increase your fluid intake.

In my experience, food intolerances (at least those that have not been detected) play a pivotal role in diverticula disease. For more on food intolerances, see Chapter 6 page 30.

Natural supports include:

- **Identifying and eliminating food intolerances**
- **1 tsp slippery elm powder in a little warm water**

- Aloe vera juice
- Increasing fibre intake – try psyllium husks
- Investing in a probiotic.

Inflammatory Bowel Diseases

Ulcerative colitis and Crohn's disease fall under this category. Their symptoms are similar and can be very debilitating (don't I know it!). There is pain in the lower abdominal region, ranging from a dull dragging ache to gripping and severe. I remember not being able to stand up straight when I was having an attack. Stools are bloody and mucousy, and you may suffer both constipation and diarrhoea. The accompanying fatigue is an additional blow.

Natural supports include:

- Reducing inflammation with either turmeric or omega-3 fish oil supplements (with an EPA content of 800 mg or more)
- Identifying and eliminating food intolerances
- 1 tsp slippery elm powder in a little warm water
- Taking a probiotic containing *Saccharomyces boulardii*
- Eating/drinking fermented foods
- Taking L- glutamine.

Short Bowel Syndrome

Sometimes, inflammatory bowel conditions cause damage to the small intestine and a portion of it may need to be removed. It's also possible to be born with a short intestine.

Symptoms of short bowel syndrome include abdominal pain, diarrhoea, smelly stools, weight loss, malnutrition and fatigue. Whilst most cases are automatically treated with medications, it is possible to manage this condition with dietary changes and supplemental support.

Natural supports include:

- **Drinking fluids regularly (electrolyte drinks will help top off nutritional deficiencies)**
- **Eating small meals – avoiding gluten and dairy**
- **Taking L-glutamine**
- **Taking a probiotic containing *Lactobacillus acidophilus***
- **Including fermented food in your diet.**

Small Intestine Bacterial Overgrowth (SIBO)

This condition arises due to too many bacteria accumulating in the wrong place. Symptoms very much mirror other digestive disorders: bloating, gas, nausea, heartburn, lower abdominal pain, erratic stools and bad breath. Hmmm. So how do you know you have it? Fortunately, there is a simple breath test that measures the amount of hydrogen or methane in your breath after drinking a water and glucose mixture. A high level indicates bacterial overgrowth in your small intestine. Other tests include the invasive jejunal aspiration test (using an endoscopy to take a sample from the small intestine to cultivate and test) and the trialling of specific medications, evaluating their impact.

Natural supports include:

- A probiotic containing *Saccharomyces boulardii* (a yeast-based strain ideal for SIBO)
- Grapefruit seed extract
- Olive leaf extract
- Pau d'arco
- Garlic.

Parasites

Intestinal parasites produce a variety of uncomfortable digestive symptoms and usually cause weakness, loss of appetite, weight loss and anaemia. They can enter the body through dirty water, uncooked meat and poor hygiene habits. Faecal testing can identify the species present.

Natural supports include:

- Observing hygiene – especially hand washing
- Drinking clean water regularly throughout the day
- Eating raw garlic
- Taking a berberine supplement
- Eating papaya seeds (mix with Manuka honey, if possible, for extra benefits)
- Adding pumpkin seeds to breakfast, smoothies and salads.

Chapter 2

Hormone-related Disorders

Goitre

If your thyroid is not producing sufficient thyroid hormones (see Hypothyroidism below) it becomes bigger. An enlarged thyroid is known as a goitre. There are certain foods that contain what are known as 'goitrogens', and they affect thyroid function and/or thyroid medication because they affect iodine levels and block the activity of a thyroid enzyme.

You should avoid, or at least limit, your intake of the following:

- Broccoli (especially raw)
- Cauliflower (especially raw)
- Peaches
- Soy foods (tofu, chickpeas, hummus, tempeh, soy milk, etc.)
- Brussel sprouts
- Kale
- Peanuts
- Spinach
- Cabbage (especially raw – e.g. coleslaw)
- Millet
- Radishes
- Strawberries.

A healthy thyroid needs iodine, selenium, folic acid and vitamin E. You can check the nutritional value of common foods on pages 174–197. If you aren't eating enough foods rich in nutrients to support your thyroid, it's worth considering supplements.

Hypothyroidism (Underactive Thyroid)

This must be one of the most common issues I see amongst my female clients, and one that can easily be addressed. The thyroid gland is a small butterfly-shaped gland at the front of the neck. An underactive thyroid arises when the thyroid gland does not release enough of the two main hormones it produces: T3 (triiodothyronine) and T4 (thyroxine).

Common signs of hypothyroidism are tiredness, weight gain and low moods. Key nutrients to support the thyroid are selenium and iodine, and increasing intake of these goes a long way to addressing the issue and can often negate the use of medication. Always know your blood test results if you have been/are taking medication. See Appendix 2, pages 204–205 for what to look for.

Natural supports include[1]:

- Eating two Brazil nuts a day (your daily selenium requirement)
- Taking iodine drops (250–350 mcg a day)
- Adding spirulina to smoothies
- Snacking on dried apricots (4–5 a day)
- Increasing your zinc intake (try oily fish, pumpkin seeds, chickpeas and lentils).

1. Not if taking thyroid medication.

Levothyroxine

This is the most common medication prescribed for an underactive thyroid. Whilst taking it, you should try to avoid foods that block the use of iodine – see the list under Goitre above. At the same time, you can naturally support your thyroid by eating foods rich in iodine, selenium, folic acid and vitamin E.

To help Levothyroxine work more effectively, take it well away from food (at least three hours before or after) to ensure full absorption of the medication. If you take iron and calcium supplements as well as this medication, leave at least 4 hours between each. Steer clear of decongestants too.

NB: Taking levothyroxine over long periods of time may cause bone loss.

Hashimoto's Disease

This is the most common cause for hypothyroidism. It's an autoimmune condition in which antibodies from your immune system attack the thyroid. Therefore, just as with any other autoimmune condition, addressing inflammation by avoiding the nightshade family of vegetables (including tomatoes, sweet peppers/capsicums, aubergines/eggplant and potatoes) and taking natural anti-inflammatories such as turmeric/curcumin and omega-3 fish oil (with an EPA content above 600 mg) goes a long way to keeping symptoms at bay.

Hyperthyroidism (Overactive Thyroid)

Graves' Disease

This is the most common cause of *hyper*thyroidism in the UK. Like Hashimoto's, it's an autoimmune disease. In Graves' disease, the antibodies mimic the activity of TSH (thyroid stimulating hormone) causing imbalances that lead to symptoms of hyperthyroidism, which include weight loss, anxiety, muscle weakness and heat intolerance. It's common to be referred for a TRab (Thyrotropin Receptor antibodies test) to establish if Grave's disease is present.

About 1 in 25 people with Graves' disease also develop thyroid eye disease, called Graves' ophthalmopathy. This is when the muscles in your eyes and the surrounding tissue swell up, giving your eyes a bulging appearance. Your eyes may become red and puffy and, occasionally, it can lead to double vision or limited movement of your eyeball.

Your doctor may prescribe anti-thyroid medicines such as carbimazole and propylthiouracil, to reduce the production of thyroid hormones. However, over time, anti-thyroid medicines can lead to hypothyroidism (an underactive thyroid), so you will need regular blood tests to monitor whether you are taking the correct dose. Remember to ask for copies of any blood test results so that you can track what's happening and become proactive rather than reactive.

Natural supports include:

- Avoiding dairy products (for Grave's Disease)
- L-Carnitine supplement to increase TSH
- Co-enzyme Q10 (levels are lower with hyperthyroidism)
- Avoiding nightshades (e.g. tomatoes, potatoes, sweet peppers/capsicums, aubergines/eggplant)
- Eating broccoli.

Diabetes

Diabetes occurs when your pancreas is unable to produce sufficient insulin to cope with the amount of glucose (sugar) in your blood; or when blood sugars fall too low and glucagon is released. It is therefore crucial to your health that you keep your blood sugars in the normal range to prevent diabetes-related health conditions. Fortunately, this condition can be very well managed (and even reversed) with a change of lifestyle and healthy eating.

Diabetes means you are more vulnerable to liver disease. You should therefore avoid processed food as much as possible to avoid putting your liver under unnecessary strain. Processed food is full of additives, colourings and preservatives that increase the amount of toxins your liver has to filter.

Natural supports include:

- Eat plenty of fresh fruit and vegetables and avoid ready meals, packets and tinned food
- You will also need to control the amount of carbohydrates and sugars you have, but you do not have to eliminate them altogether.

The Glycaemic Index measures the speed at which carbohydrates break down into sugar in our bodies. Low GI foods are digested slowly, keep you feeling fuller for longer and help to keep your blood glucose levels even.

Low GI Foods (0–55)	Moderate GI Foods (55–70)	High GI Foods (70–100)
All bran	Shredded wheat	Cornflakes
Buckwheat	Couscous	Tapioca
Brown rice	Basmati rice	Short grain white rice
Wholegrain bread	Pita bread	French bread

Low GI Foods (0–55)	Moderate GI Foods (55–70)	High GI Foods (70–100)
Pasta	New potatoes	Baked/mashed potatoes
Grapefruit	Bananas	Dates
Lentils	Sultanas	Parsnips
Broccoli	Beetroot	Pumpkin
Peanuts	Muesli bars	Honey
Oats	Rice bubbles	Jelly beans

Metformin

Metformin is a medication often prescribed to help control Type 2 diabetes, but it has been shown to decrease cognitive performance. Researchers suggested that taking calcium and B12 supplements may help alleviate metformin-induced B12 deficiency and lead to better cognitive outcomes. Metformin also interferes with magnesium levels, so if you've noticed a change in your bowel movements (especially an urgency to go) since taking it or increasing the dose, consider speaking with your doctor to have the dose adjusted.

More information can be found in my Handy Book of Facts on Diabetes (available via www.alisoncowell.com)

Pre-Menstrual Tension (PMS/PMT)

PMS is a combination of physical and emotional symptoms that occur in the days following ovulation and leading up to a period. Physical symptoms can include bloating, sore breasts, changes in bowel movements, headaches and cramps; emotional symptoms include low moods, anxiety, irritability, insomnia, low libido, lack of concentration and appetite changes.

Whilst it's common for women to experience a variety of these symptoms, if they are continually severe and prolonged, then it goes beyond PMS and is likely *Premenstrual Dysphoric Disorder* (PDD).

Natural supports include:

- Calcium
- Chaste tree
- Gingko Biloba
- Vitamin B6
- Evening Primrose Oil
- Magnesium.

Polycystic Ovary Syndrome (PCOS)

PCOS symptoms are varied and quite obscure, which is why it often goes undiagnosed.

Common symptoms include:

- Acne
- Irregular periods
- Insulin resistance
- Increased facial and body hair
- Intolerance to heat/hot weather
- Weight gain

On the latter point, if weight gain is a symptom for you (it isn't for everyone), then reducing your carbohydrate intake at night will help.

Foods to include	Foods to avoid
Mostly low Glycaemic Index (GI) foods	Alcohol
Plenty of fresh 'low sugar' fruit (e.g.-apples oranges, mandarins)	Caffeine
Non-starchy vegetables (e.g. carrots, cauliflower, broccoli, spinach)	Processed foods (i.e. lots of additives, preservatives and colourings)
Fish – at least 3 times a week	High-fat foods
Whole grains, seeds and nuts	Sugary foods, including honey and syrup
Watercress in your salads	Food additive 320 (butylated hydroxyanisole)
Flax seeds	

Natural supports include:

Helpful supplements

- Zinc (15 mg)
- Chromium (500 mg)
- Omega-3 (with at least 800 mg of both EPA and DHA)
- Inositol (1000 mg)
- Magnesium (500 mg)
- Vitamin B6 (100 mg)
- Vitamin B12 (100 mcg)

Beneficial herbs

- Kava kava
- Siberian ginseng
- Bladderwrack
- St John's Wort (but not if you are taking antidepressants or oral contraceptives).

Endometriosis

Endometriosis is the abnormal growth of cells that usually form in the lining of the uterus. Instead of being expelled in a menstrual flow, these tissues remain in the body and can attach themselves to other organs, including the lower abdomen and bowel. The ensuing result can lead to pain and inflammation.

Recent research (*American Journal of Obstetrics & Gynaecology, 2017*) suggests probiotics may help with prevention and/or management. Whilst there is no 'cure' for this condition, adjustments to your diet can make a tremendous difference and even allow you to live in remission of the symptoms.

Foods to include	Food to avoid
Broccoli	Red meat
Cauliflower	Ham (sodium nitrate content)
Nuts – especially almonds and cashew nuts	High sugar foods
Olives	High 'bad' fat foods
Avocados	Dairy products
Chia seeds	Alcohol

Foods to include	Foods to avoid
Lemons	Nightshades (potatoes, tomatoes, sweet peppers/capsicums, aubergines/eggplant, chillies)
Oily fish (salmon, tuna, sardines, etc.)	Pickles
Soy foods	Cheese
Fermented foods (kombucha, kefir, kimchi)	Refined carbohydrates (white flour, white rice, etc.)

Drinking herbal teas can help. Try red raspberry leaf, sage or chasteberry.

Other helpful drinks include:

- Apple cider vinegar – 2 tsps in a glass of water
- Dandelion or nettle tea.

Beneficial supplements include:

- Probiotics
- Vitamin B5 and B6 (at least 100 mg of each)
- Vitamin E
- Turmeric (or curcumin)
- DIM (diindolylmethane)
- Magnesium
- Omega-3 (with an EPA content of at least 600 mg)
- Iron (if heavy menstrual blood loss)
- Iodine.

Infertility

Whilst everyone is different, the following principles are a helpful guide to those having difficulty conceiving:

Both partners:

- Avoid caffeine and alcohol and keep weight within a healthy range
- Invest in a probiotic (healthy bacteria) supplement or eat fermented food every day
- Identify food intolerances
- Check for presence of candida albicans (a pathogenic yeast)
- Deal with any stresses in your life as best you can. Learn how to relax and breathe deeply through activities such as yoga, Pilates and qigong. Listen to relaxation tapes as you go to bed
- Don't smoke
- Eat a well-balanced diet that includes plenty of fresh, natural food (avoiding preservatives and additives as much as possible)
- Take apple cider vinegar.

Girls	Guys
Boost your immune system. If your immune system is weak, your body will 'protect' you by avoiding pregnancy. In addition to the herbs below, take plenty of fresh garlic whenever you can.	Wear loose fitting clothes and keep cool.
Supplements: • Zinc • Vitamin E • Iron • Vitamin B6 • Evening primrose oil • Omega-3 fish oil • Black cohosh • Red raspberry leaf (but stop taking during the first half of your pregnancy) • Donq quai • Probiotics	**Supplements:** • Zinc – improve quality and quantity of sperm and increase testosterone levels • Vitamin C – another boost for healthy sperm • Vitamin E • Astragalus • Arginine • Probiotics

It helps to know what's going on in your body, so ask for copies of any blood tests to identify areas needing attention or support.

Apart from nutrition, there are complementary therapies that can help maximize your chances of pregnancy, including chiropractic, reflexology, aromatherapy and acupuncture.

Menopause

Firstly, I need to acknowledge that this is not a 'health issue', but rather a naturally occurring event that every female will experience.

Many women expect to have an awful time due to the conversations and perceptions that have gone before. For instance there's a common shared image entitled 'The Seven Dwarves of Menopause' with little figures called 'itchy, bitchy, sweaty, sleepy, bloated, forgetful and psycho'! Little wonder then that the first signs of menopause approaching can cause many women to rush off for hormone replacement therapy before allowing their bodies to naturally deal with the changing hormones in their bodies.

Prior to menopause itself is the transitional stage known as perimenopause, or pre-menopause. This is when oestrogen levels begin to drop but menstruation is still occurring. You might experience irritability, loss of libido, mood swings, irregular periods and night sweats (or you might not). I've included an oestrogen score chart in Appendix 7, page 216 if you're keen to assess yourself.

It's easy to focus on the main hormones of oestrogen, progesterone and testosterone at this time. However, other hormones also need to be acknowledged, including adrenalin and cortisol. When I'm dealing with anyone in the perimenopausal stage, I always make sure that we get blood tests looking at *all* the hormonal markers, which in turn allows us to focus on the areas that need support, not just the obvious.

Menopause itself is the cessation of menstrual periods for over 1 year. This generally happens between the ages of 45 and 55 years old. Nutritious food, quality sleep and exercise are more important than ever.

I have listed some helpful supplements and herbs that will help balance hormones, and also some that support bone health because bone loss is more prevalent in post-menopausal women. Calcium levels deplete as you hit menopause, so it's important to have magnesium and calcium to lower your risk of conditions such as osteoporosis and osteoarthritis as you age. That's where weight-bearing exercise is also important at this time.

Natural supports include:

- A magnesium, calcium and vitamin D combo
- Evening primrose oil
- Omega-3
- Maca powder (I'm a real fan of this!)
- Red clover
- Sage
- Chaste tree.

Prostate health

The prostate gland is part of the male reproductive system and sits just below the bladder. It plays a pivotal role in the production of seminal fluid. It's important to look after prostate health because issues such as prostatitis and cancer often present with seemingly insignificant or unrelated symptoms, including poor bladder control or difficulty urinating.

Prostatitis is a common swelling or inflammation of the prostate, often affecting younger men. An enlarged prostate or benign prostatic hypertrophy (BPH) generally affects older men.

Natural supports include:

- Two Brazil nuts a day – for selenium
- Oily fish
- Avocados
- Pomegranates/pomegranate juice.

Prostate Cancer

Research has proven that tumours thrive in an acidic environment so have apple cider vinegar to alkalise your system (2 tsps in a glass of water).

Drink a glass of vegetable juice a day to help fight free radicals. A plant-based diet has been proven to beneficial for prostate health and this is a great way to boost your intake.

Eat less polyunsaturated fat (the kind often found in baked and fried goods) and reduce your intake of red meat.

Green tea and oolong tea may help stop progression of prostate cancer according to studies in India in 2009.

Lycopene (an antioxidant found in foods such as broccoli and tomatoes) may prohibit the growth of prostate cancer cells. Eating tomatoes and broccoli together can maximize their protective effect against prostate cancer, according to a study published by Cancer Research. Whilst these two vegetables are known for their cancer-fighting properties, the research concluded that used together they are more effective in shrinking prostate tumours. Add them to stir frys and salads.

Eating just one serving or more of broccoli and cauliflower a week may reduce risk of prostate cancer by up to 45 percent, according to a study published in the August 2007 issue of Journal of the National Cancer Institute.

Selenium is another important ally. Just two Brazil nuts will provide your daily intake, so get nibbling!

Fish omega-3 may decrease the spread of prostate cancer by about 43 percent, according to Swedish researchers. Another study by the British Journal of Cancer, found that the type of fatty acids determines how they influence the risk of metastatic prostate cancer. The UK researchers found omega-3 fatty acids inhibit proliferation of prostate cancer cells. If you are not a fan of salmon or other oily fish look for a quality supplement such as Ethical Nutrients Hi-Strength liquid fish oil. (Reports in 2013 suggesting an increased risk of prostate cancer if taking omega-3 have been dismissed.)

Drinking pomegranate juice may help slow the growth of prostate cancer, suggests a small study published in Clinical Cancer Research. The study found it took a longer time for men who drank pomegranate juice to double PSA in their blood. PSA is a protein marker indicating the presence of prostate cancer. As always, get to know your numbers when you have a blood test so you can take control and ask questions at the right time. I had a client, a very fit and healthy 70 year old with no health issues, who went for regular blood tests every year as part of his annual check-up, and PSA was included. It had been progressively increasing but his doctor hadn't picked it up until it was way outside the normal range. Sadly, cancer had developed, but it could and should have been identified much sooner.

Vitamin E has also been shown to have positive impact on prostate health. Add avocados to your salads for an easy boost of this vitamin.

Chapter 3

Nervous System Disorders

Migraines

There is a HUGE distinction between a very bad headache and a migraine – ask any sufferer. Migraines are debilitating and exhausting, and a serious attack can lead to vertigo, vomiting and even paralysis.

Causes include:

- Food triggers, including chocolate, cheese, alcohol and caffeine
- Magnesium deficiency – magnesium helps to dilate blood vessels throughout the body, so a lack of it leads to constriction of the vessels. Constricted vessels in the head contribute to the throbbing sensation most sufferers experience
- Hormones – migraines are more common in women due to the drop in oestrogen levels
- Tyramine – an amino acid that occurs in many foods including avocados, bananas, coconuts, corned beef, pork and peanuts. Whilst the body should metabolise tyramine, some systems struggle and this can lead to health conditions including migraines, burning mouth and tongue, high blood pressure and panic attacks (see Appendix 3, page 196)
- Low vitamin D

- Low vitamin B2 – found in organ meats, almonds, mushrooms and whole grains, this energy-boosting vitamin can help prevent migraines

- MSG (monosodium glutamate – food additive 621) can cause headaches, water retention and respiratory problems. It's in many processed foods, including potato chips, but most commonly in Chinese foods and sauces, so limit your intake of these.

Natural remedies:

- Co-enzyme Q10. This naturally occurring chemical is found in foods such as broccoli, kumara, spinach, soy foods, oily fish and most meat – but note that frying reduces CoQ10 levels. Supplements containing at least 300 mg will help prevent migraines (and help address other health conditions, including cholesterol, heart conditions and chronic fatigue)

- Omega-3. Oily fish are high in omega-3 and research has shown a positive effect of omega-3 on migraines, so include salmon, mackerel and sardines in your diet whenever you can

- Water is a must to keep the body hydrated and migraines at bay. Pure, filtered water should be sipped throughout the day

- Lavender oil has been proven to have calming and healing effects for treating headaches and migraines. Apply some to your temples and also on your pillow before you go to sleep at night.

Depression

According to statistics, up to 20% of New Zealanders are affected by depression at some time in their lives, with a staggering 1 in 5 young people being diagnosed each year. Pacific youngsters are twice as likely to suffer with depression or make suicide attempts as the rest of the population. In the UK, statistics are conflicting and confusing depending on the information source. That said, the trend appears to be showing a slight increase in the number of reported cases. *However, this could be the tip of the ice-berg because many people suffer in silence, feeling helpless, hopeless and even embarrassed to admit they have a problem.*

Depression is more than having an off day or feeling low now and then (that would account for most of us!).

Signs of depression in an individual include:

- **Nothing stimulates or excites them**
- **Everyday tasks seem too much to bear and everything becomes an effort**
- **They feel worthless or a burden**
- **They are tearful all the time**
- **They don't care about their appearance or the state of their home**
- **They don't want to go out**
- **Becoming unreasonable with family and friends.**

If symptoms like these persist for more than 2 weeks, it's likely depression. Once a diagnosis is made, the common solution is to prescribe antidepressants. However, the relationship between mood and food has been extensively researched and documented, and there are many ways for an individual to take back control of their lives by eating the right food, and therefore possibly avoiding the need to medicate.

In the UK I have been delivering a series of workshops on mood and food. It's been wonderful to hear afterwards from those who have attended, and who tell me that by making the suggested changes to their diets they noticed positive impacts on their mood, behaviour and sleep patterns.

One of the most revealing, and quite shocking, points that I make is how the side effects of everyday medications can be responsible for causing so many mood issues. Here are some examples.

Asthma

Prednisone: severe depression, personality changes, extreme sadness.

Hypo (underactive) Thyroid

Levothyroxine: anxiety, depression, sleep disruption.

Diabetes

Metformin: panic attacks, anxiety, depression.

High Cholesterol

Atorvastatin, Simvastatin: nightmares, nervousness, depression.

Now, just suppose that you were asthmatic, with high cholesterol and diabetes? You might soon find that you were taking an antidepressant to complement your medicine collection. Who would be making the link?

Knowledge is power, so check the side effects of any medications you're taking. I know I'm like a broken record when it comes to that message, but if you sat in my seat and saw the implications as often as I do, you'd surely be the same!

Natural remedies:

We need magnesium, omega-3 and B vitamins to make 'happy' brain chemicals like noradrenalin and dopamine. To produce serotonin (perhaps the best-known brain chemical) we require essential amino acids tryptophan and methionine. Methionine is broken down in the liver to produce a sub-amino acid called S-adenosylmethionine (SAM-e for short!), whilst tryptophan is a precursor for serotonin. Nutritional deficiencies most commonly arise due to food intolerances. In fact, lactose (and fructose) intolerance inhibits the absorption of tryptophan.

Given that 90% of serotonin is produced and absorbed in the gut, a healthy digestive system is essential to keep depression at bay.

The following can help*:

Foods to include	Supplements
Oats	Probiotic containing the strains *Lacto-bacillus helveticus and rhamnosus*
Barley	B vitamin complex
Bananas	Omega-3
Tuna, salmon and snapper	Magnesium
Probiotic yoghurt	5-HTP (5 hydroxy-tryptophan) St. John's Wort

See Appendix 5 for meal ideas.

* *NB: The above may not be suitable for everyone depending on current health, existing medications, food intolerances and whether pregnant.*

Did you know?

Smiling boosts your immune system and helps prolong your life. In fact, the broader your smile and the deeper the creases around your eyes when you grin, the longer you are likely to live, according to a study published in *Psychological Science*. So, what are you waiting for? Flash those pearly whites right now!

Anxiety

It's normal to feel anxious or worried in certain situations. In fact, it would be worrying if you didn't! It's part of our human 'fight or flight' response. When we believe we are in danger, our brains release a powerful chemical called adrenocorticotropic hormone (ACTH).

However, if the feeling of unease or panic is persistent and begins to impact on your daily life and/or sleep pattern then it indicates a malfunction of this fight or flight response.

Natural solutions are the same as those suggested for adrenal fatigue on page 144.

Insomnia

There are no hard and fast rules about how much sleep is enough because we are all different. Even our own sleep patterns change as we age. However, whilst one or two sleepless nights might cause irritability and tiredness the following day, ongoing sleeplessness can lead to chronic bouts of fatigue, depression and a deterioration in overall performance. It can also signify an underlying medical condition that needs to be addressed, which is why a personal consultation is highly recommended.

I've found that many of my clients who work shifts (especially night shifts) have sleep issues. I've prepared a fact sheet (see Appendix 6, page 214) with some helpful tips on this subject.

Nutritionally, there are many nutrients that can help, including:

- Magnesium – encourages melatonin production and helps prevent restless legs during the night
- Calcium – has a calming effect on the body
- Vitamin B6 (pyridoxine) – can aid hormonal sleep disturbances, relieve stress and promote REM (Rapid Eye Movement) sleep
- Vitamin B3 (niacin) – particularly helpful when insomnia is connected with depression
- 5-HTP (5-hydroxy-tryptophan) – tryptophan is a sleep promoting chemical and also an anti-stress support. NB: Not be taken if you are taking antidepressants
- Iodine – will support your adrenal glands (and they need all the help they can get in this busy world!) NB: Not to be taken if you have a thyroid condition without first checking with your healthcare provider.

Foods that can help sleep: (food intolerances excepted)

- Cherries, walnuts, flax seed, tomatoes, figs, dates, red and orange capsicums/sweet peppers, bananas, nuts, seeds, honey, eggs, dairy products (especially yoghurt) and turkey
- Herbal teas such as chamomile, kava kava, lemon balm.

Foods that can hinder sleep:

- Alcohol, spicy foods, high fat foods, coffee, bacon, ham, and dark chocolate
- Do not eat a large evening meal within two hours of bedtime.

Eye Health

Eyes are part of the sensory nervous system. There are a number of conditions that affect eye health, from minor annoyances such as blepharitis and styes to more serious and debilitating conditions such as cataracts and macular degeneration. Whilst there are specific treatments to address each of these conditions, there are nutrients that will support, protect and even improve eye health.

Beta-carotene

The body converts beta-carotene to vitamin A, and this has been scientifically proven to reduce the risk of cataracts and macular degeneration, support the surface of the eye (the cornea), protect the mucous membrane (preventing dryness) and provide a barrier for bacteria and viruses. Any orange-coloured fruits and veg will contain this important compound (carrots being an obvious example!).

Red-carotene

Found in red-coloured foods such as tomatoes, beetroot, etc.; contains anti-oxidants that help support vision and keep free radicals at bay.

Lutein

Found in dark green leafy vegetables such as spinach and kale; one of the best-known eye-protecting antioxidants, particularly good for retina health. Sweetcorn, peas and broccoli also contain large amounts of lutein.

Zeaxanthin

Found in dark leafy vegetables, paprika and saffron. It supports central macula function.

Omega-3 Essential Fatty Acids

Found in oily fish such as salmon, tuna and mackerel; can reduce underlying inflammation and help prevent dry eyes.

Chapter 4

Skin and Hair Disorders

The Skin

Did you know that your skin is the largest organ of your body? It consists of three layers: the epidermis on the outside, the dermis in the middle and the hypodermis at the base. Skin cells grow from the inside out, so whilst you can certainly feed it from the outside in, you must ensure the new developing cells have all the right nutrients to keep them as healthy as possible.

Top nutrients include zinc; vitamins A, C and E; omega-3 and, naturally, lots of water! It's also useful to invest in a probiotic containing the *Lactobacillus rhamnosus* (GG) strain. There is an absolute link between a healthy gut and healthy skin.

As you can imagine, people with skin issues feature in large numbers on my database. It can be distressing and, at times, debilitating.

Case Study

Hannah, a 6-month-old baby, was one of my clients. So severe was the eczema on her face, it was like a hard mask, and the poor little thing couldn't laugh or cry because it was too painful. Her Mum had taken her off dairy and had switched to soy milk, but the eczema didn't improve. When I tested Hannah, it transpired that she was more intolerant to soy than to dairy and she also had an issue with eggs. I'll never forget when I saw her for her review just 4 weeks later, with beautiful skin and a beaming smile.

Case Study

Chris, a taxi driver, had a severe form of eczema and an autoimmune condition called Grover's Disease, which affects the skin. Chris's hands were so affected that he couldn't hold the steering wheel of his car anymore, threatening his livelihood. Again, I identified his food intolerances, adjusted his diet, recommended the correct supplements for him and in a very short time, his hands were as supple as mine.

Rashes

Rashes can be itchy, raised, smooth, pale coloured, fierce and appear anywhere on your body.

There are a host of potential reasons for skin rashes and there is a process to go through to determine each individual cause. Most common causes are irritants (harsh deodorants, perfumes, fabric conditioners, etc.), pollutants (including air-borne chemicals such as pesticides used in farms and orchards, and 'insect killer' sprays), fungal infections (too many harmful yeasts in your system), the side-effects of medications and, of course, food. It is helpful to keep a food and symptom diary to help identify culprits (see Appendix 9, pages 220–221) and/or consider a food intolerance test.

A persistent rash and/or one that appears in the same place can sometimes be a sign of a more serious health condition. A butterfly rash on the face, for example, may be an indication of Lupus (an autoimmune condition) or perhaps a blood disorder. They need to be taken seriously and it is wise to ask for a blood test.

Other tests that may be performed are biopsies:

- **Skin biopsy – removing skin cells or skin samples**
- **Shave biopsy – removing the top layer of the skin (epidermis)**
- **Punch biopsy – removing a small section of skin using a small circular tool**
- **Excisional biopsy – removing an entire portion of skin.**

Of course, the rest of your health needs to be assessed in conjunction with any rash. If there is a sudden deterioration in health accompanied by a rash, seek advice immediately. Conditions such as meningitis require prompt intervention.

Case Study

A worried son asked me to visit his elderly mother, Eileen, in a retirement village. "She has an annoying rash that won't go away" he told me, "and after hearing you speak recently, I think it could be due to a food intolerance". I went to see Eileen and was immediately struck by the severity of the rash. "Annoying?" This rash was utterly torturous for poor Eileen. She was clawing at her skin so much that carers had to come in every morning to change the sheets on her bed and apply new dressings to all the bleeding parts of her skin (she looked like a Mummy!) I had never seen a food intolerance cause such an extreme reaction and, although I didn't rule it out, I wasn't convinced food was the culprit. I asked Eileen how long she had been suffering with the rash, and she was quite specific. "Seems everything went downhill the day I turned 84. Perhaps it's psychological, but I haven't felt right since. My skin is only one problem I have". Eileen had turned 84 eight months prior to my visit, so the poor woman had been suffering since then.

I dug deeper. Eileen told me that on her 84th birthday she had undergone an extensive health check and was advised to take various medications afterwards. I asked to see all of them, *together with any supplements she was taking. She had so many, she couldn't fit them all on her table!*

I was familiar with most (same old 'solutions' for high blood pressure, cholesterol, diabetes, insomnia, indigestion and depression), including a popular choice for managing osteoarthritis (a deteriorating bone condition). I knew that most of the medications had side effects, especially the one for osteoarthritis, which carried an explicit warning that if a skin rash appeared, the medication should be stopped. I pointed it out to Eileen and mentioned the timing. I suggested she stop the medication and notice what happened. "Oh no dear, I couldn't do that..." she said as she scratched yet another wound in her skin, "...my doctor said I had to take them for my bones". I tried to convince Eileen that her bones wouldn't crumble in a week, and that's all we would need to see if the medication was causing her skin issue. However, she was reluctant to alter anything.

Frustrated, I went back to her son and told him my thoughts. He agreed that I should write to Eileen's doctor, show photographs of the skin, together with the data sheet from the medication, and ask if the doctor would consent to her stopping the tablets, if only temporarily. A curt note came back basically telling me that I was not a doctor, I should not interfere, and that this medication had been prescribed safely to many patients, including those in the same retirement village as Eileen, and had never caused a problem. So no, thank you very much, she would not be telling Eileen to stop.

Eileen stuck by her doctor's word and I could do no more than offer suggestions to naturally treat and heal her skin, knowing full well that I wasn't tackling the cause.

A few weeks later, I was giving a presentation to Age Concern and Eileen was in the audience. I only knew she was there because there was a slight commotion following her blood seeping through her bandages onto the blouse of the person sitting next to her in the audience! I took the opportunity to catch up with her afterwards. She looked and felt miserable. I asked what further action had been taken to get to the root of her skin problem. Nothing had. Fortunately, Eileen's son was with her, so I ran through a number of suggestions he could follow up, including referral to a dermatologist.

Four months later, I had a lovely letter from Eileen's son letting me know that he had taken the matter further as suggested. The dermatologist was appalled at the state of Eileen's skin, and that she had suffered for so long. Infections were setting in (but fear not, dear reader, there were a raft of antibiotics prescribed for those ... sigh) and her scabs were not healing. He immediately linked the symptoms to the medication and Eileen stopped taking the tablets.

Her son was writing to let me know that Eileen had died. She had end-stage kidney disease. I was not surprised. If her body was screaming so obviously on the outside, I could only imagine the internal struggle going on with her liver and kidneys trying to cope with such toxicity.

I think of Eileen very often. It's because of people like her that I have this passion to continue raising awareness of our body's inbuilt alarm systems, and how we should not ignore them.

Eczema

Eczema is itchy, dry, rough, flaky, inflamed and irritated skin. It often comes and goes and can occur anywhere but usually affects the arms and legs. There are various types including discoid, pompholyx and seborrheic, but most common is atopic. Increasing your intake of omega-3 through oily fish or supplementation is beneficial, together with a probiotic containing *Lactobacillus rhamnosus*. Eliminating dairy and gluten has proven benefits, but I recommend you have a full food intolerance test to establish your personal culprits!

Dermatitis

Dermatitis usually arises after contact with substances containing acid or alkaline materials such as soaps and detergents, fabric softeners, solvents or other chemicals. Because it presents similar to eczema, with dry, itchy inflamed skin, it is often misdiagnosed. Patch testing can help.

Welts/wheals/hives/urticaria

Welts, wheals, hives and urticaria are raised sections of skin that are irritated and somewhat elevated in comparison with the surrounding skin area. Their appearance is anywhere from pale purple to fiery red in colour. Often the area is tender to the touch and may also be itchy.

Case Study

Perhaps one of the worst cases I have seen was Bryony (it was not long before I started this book in fact). Bryony came to see me for digestive problems, but it was painfully obvious that she was having extreme issues with her skin – huge, large, painful welts that looked as though she had been burnt with acid. Years of suffering had left her with scars. When I mentioned them, she simply shrugged – she *had resigned herself to the fact that it was "just one of those things". She had seen specialists, dermatologists, naturopaths, a dietician and no-one had been able to help, other than provide her with harsh steroid creams, antibiotics and painkillers. At one point she was on methotrexate, a medication used for cancer patients.*

During my consultations, I always ask if any organs have been removed, because it matters if part of your engine is missing!

Of course, you can live without tonsils, appendix, gall bladder, etc., but there is a consequence to them going. Bryony recalled that her appendix had burst in 2003, some 14 years ago. I could see the lights coming on as we spoke ... the welts had started to appear shortly after that time. We investigated the medications and anaesthetics used and discovered that they were high in salicylates. Salicylates are natural chemicals found in many plants and, although natural, they can cause welts in those who are sensitive (they can also cause ADHD).

To prove the theory that Bryony had indeed had an extreme reaction to the medication used at the time and was now highly sensitive to any salicylates, I did a hair analysis test. I was not surprised when it came back showing huge reactions to every single high salicylate on the chart! Following a low salicylate diet, Bryony noticed results almost from day one. Her digestive health, which was why she'd come along in the first place, also greatly improved.

You'll find a list of salicylates in Appendix 5, pages 210–213.

Acne

Commonly the bane of most teenagers, this annoying skin condition is usually connected with hormonal changes or imbalances.

If circulatory and excretory functions are not working efficiently, toxins will find the next easiest route out – and that's through your skin. Boosting both functions is therefore helpful to having nice, clear skin.

Natural remedies include:

- Zinc, zinc, zinc! If supplementing, look for around 40–45 mg a day
- Probiotics – look for *Bifidobacterium lactis* and *rhamnosus LGG* in particular
- Cleansing teas for liver and kidneys
- For adult acne, try vitamins B6, B2 and chromium (for insulin resistance where Polycystic Ovary Syndrome is present)
- Tea tree oil applied externally is antiseptic and healing. *Dilute it with a carrier oil (such as olive oil or coconut oil) before applying.*

Psoriasis

Psoriasis is a hereditary, chronic inflammatory skin condition, aggravated by a build-up of toxins in your system. When your body cannot eliminate those toxins through the normal route, it tries to dispose of them through your skin. Eating foods with essential fatty acids and anti-inflammatory properties will help. Research has also suggested that reducing the amount of meat protein in your diet can help this condition. Ultraviolet light is beneficial, as is bathing in Epsom salts.

You should avoid:

- Acidic foods (most citrus fruits, tomatoes, etc.)
- Sugar
- Pickled and smoked foods
- Alcohol
- All foods from the nightshade family (eggplant/aubergine, white potatoes, sweet peppers/capsicums, etc.)
- Fried foods, refined foods and salt
- Processed foods with coconut oil and palm oil
- Carbonated drinks

Keeping to a largely alkaline diet will help prevent flare-ups of this condition.

Rosacea

Rosacea is linked to *Helicobacter pylori* (*H. Pylori* – a bacteria that can be present in your gut, causing infection) and is aggravated by alcohol, smoking and poor food choices. Having SIBO (Small Intestinal Bacterial Overgrowth) is also a factor.

Lichen sclerosus

This is a chronic inflammatory skin condition that can affect any part of the body. Sometimes called white spot disease, it presents with white patches on the skin and affects mostly females, usually over the age of 50. That said, the youngest client I ever saw with this condition was a 5-year-old little girl. She was very distressed because the affected skin can become tight and itchy. Given that the most common sites are the genitals and anus, you can imagine how uncomfortable this poor wee girl was. She had developed constipation, a common side effect, and was utterly miserable. Like other autoimmune conditions, the trigger for it is not clear, although it does seem more prevalent in those who already have an existing autoimmune condition.

Natural remedies include:

- Apple cider vinegar – apply a diluted solution on to affected areas
- Lavender oil – dilute with a carrier oil if particularly sensitive
- Caster oil
- Coconut oil (notice an oil theme here?!)
- Bathing in Epsom salts (avoiding perfumes and soaps)
- Zinc supplements
- Probiotics containing the species *Lactobacillus rhamnosus*
- Omega-3 fish oil with high (at least 600 mg) EPA.

Cellulite

This is the bane of many of us! Cellulite is caused by a build-up of fat underneath the skin and leads to a lumpy and dimpled effect. Massage and exercise can improve the appearance of your skin, whilst nutritionally a diet high in essential fatty acids and antioxidant minerals will help regulate the body's fat metabolism. Oily fishes, nuts and seeds are good selections in this category. Drinking lots of water will also help flush the body and remove toxins more rapidly than dieting alone.

Here are some of the most beneficial and nutrient-packed fruits and vegetables used in many 'fat-busting' juices:

- Blueberries and blackberries
- Cherries
- Mangoes
- Oranges
- Strawberries and raspberries
- Cranberries
- Grapefruit
- Apples
- Spinach
- Tomatoes
- Fennel
- Sweet peppers/capsicums
- Carrots

Some foods may make cellulite appear worse, perish the thought! The worst offenders include alcohol (which dehydrates your body), refined foods (including foods high in artificial additives and sweeteners), sodas and eating a diet overly high in animal protein.

Cellulitis

Cellulitis occurs when *Streptococcus* or *Staphylococcus* bacteria infection enters a break in the skin. This condition mainly affects older adults and occurs in the lower legs, but it can affect *anyone* and occur anywhere in the body. It can mimic other conditions, including deep vein thrombosis, so seek medical attention for a correct diagnosis if the site is painful, swollen and/or inflamed.

Foods to include	Foods to avoid
Fresh fruit and veg	Alcohol
Fish (at least 3 times a week)	Caffeine
White meat	Processed foods (i.e. lots of additives, preservatives and colourings)
	High fat foods
	Sugary foods

Helpful supplements:

- Probiotics – useful to strengthen the immune system following use of antibiotics
- Quercetin (1500 mg) – a flavonoid known to reduce lymphoedema
- Zinc (30 mg)
- Vitamin C (1000 mg).

Applied topically to the skin:[1]

- Manuka honey – healing and soothing
- Diluted tea tree oil – antifungal.

The following can also be applied directly to the skin. Available from most health food stores either in powders that can be mixed to a paste with water, or teas that can be applied to the skin on cotton wool when cool:

1. See A leg ulcer poultice on page 104.

- Fenugreek seed – anti-inflammatory and healing
- Yarrow – antibacterial and anti-inflammatory properties
- Calendula flower – anti-inflammatory.

Leg Ulcers

Amongst the most common causes for leg ulcers are poor circulation, varicose veins, diabetes and thrombophlebitis.

Foods to include	Foods to avoid
Fresh fruit and veg (try and eat as much raw food as possible)	Alcohol
Garlic and turmeric are particularly good for boosting circulation	Caffeine
Fish – at least 3 times a week	Processed foods (i.e. lots of additives, preservatives and colourings)
Lean meat	High fat foods
	Sugary foods

Helpful supplements:

- Co-enzyme Q10 (60 mg) and co-enzyme QA (amount depends on blend of the brand you buy)
- B vitamin complex (at least 100 mg of each B vitamin)
- Zinc (20 mg)
- Omega-3 (with at least 600 mg of both EPA & DHA).

Beneficial herbs:

- Alfalfa
- Red Clover
- Goldenseal.

A leg ulcer poultice

Manuka honey applied directly onto the ulcer will be healing and soothing. You can also make a poultice using dried fenugreek, flax seed and slippery elm. First, clean the area to be treated. Then crush the dried herbs together until they form a powder. Slowly add warm water (previously boiled) until the mixture becomes a thick paste. Smear onto a clean piece of muslin and gently cover the ulcer. Wrap with a cotton towel or a bandage to secure. It can be left on the leg for up to 24 hours but no longer. If you find a poultice too onerous to produce, simply mix Manuka honey with mashed avocado and apply directly to the affected area.

Melanomas

You can reduce your risk of skin melanoma by increasing your intake of co-enzyme Q10, selenium and zinc. Scientific evidence has also shown that cooked tomatoes protect the skin from the harmful ultraviolet rays of the sun, due to the powerful anticancer properties of lycopene and lutein.

Alopecia

There are many different types of alopecia, including androgenetic, cicatricial, areata, telogen effluvium, anagen effluvium, traction and trichotillomania. The most common are the first two. Tests can identify (or eliminate) which type. Causes range from harsh shampoos to the side effects of medications, to stress.

All foods with silica in them will encourage hair re-growth; cucumber, radishes, carrots, garlic, bean sprouts, onions, sesame seeds, dandelion and millet are amongst the best. Eat plenty of fresh and raw fruit, veg, nuts and seeds (intolerances permitting – walnuts have unique omega-3s that have been linked to hair regrowth). Avoid raw egg dishes (such as mayonnaise) and eliminate dairy.

Supplements to help:

- Evening primrose oil
- A good B-vitamin complex
- Zinc (I suggest 35 mg a day to stimulate cell renewal)
- Gingko biloba – stimulates the scalp in particular
- If your condition is caused by stress, try taking an adrenal support supplement (there are quite a few to choose from)
- A probiotic containing the species *Lactobacillus rhamnosus GG.*

Also, try using apple cider vinegar and sage tea externally on your head.

Chapter 5

Joint and Bone Disorders

Bones are made from living, growing tissue and are mostly comprised of collagen and calcium phosphate.

Bone remodelling happens throughout our lifetime; mature bone tissue is removed from the skeleton (known as resorption) and new bone tissue is formed (known as ossification). This ensures a healthy bone mass as we age, which is why increasing both collagen and calcium intake is particularly beneficial to protect from conditions such as osteoporosis, especially if it's already in your family.

Osteopenia

This is a condition signalling low bone mass and is often a precursor to osteoporosis. It doesn't usually cause any symptoms but, as prevention is always better than cure, keep an eye on body signals that may indicate your bones need support:

- **Your posture – are you noticing that you are stooping?**
- **Your fingernails – are they weak and brittle?**
- **Injury-prone – do your bones appear to break easily?**
- **Weak grip strength**
- **Receding gums**
- **Blood tests – they can reveal low levels of calcium and vitamin D. Your health practitioner may also check your DHEA (dehydroepiandrosterone) level and check for fluoride toxicity.**

Fortunately, when it comes to nutrition, bones respond very well and it's possible to reverse bone loss. It's understandable that most people turn to calcium as a booster for bone health, but there are equally important nutrients required including:

- Calcium
- Magnesium
- Vitamin D
- Vitamin E
- Vitamin K (K2).

Osteoporosis

Literally translated as 'porous bones', this condition develops when new bone formation doesn't keep up with old bone loss. This leaves bones weak and more liable to fracture. Like osteopenia above, it isn't painful in itself. However, the resultant change of posture as the spine succumbs, or at the site of a fracture, can cause discomfort.

Osteoarthritis

This happens through wear and tear of joints caused by the breakdown of cartilage. Cartilage is there to cushion the bones that form the joints. It not only avoids direct friction between the bones but also helps to absorb shock.

When you suffer from osteoarthritis, the bones rub together due to loss of cartilage and eventually the bone health and strength deteriorates and fluid accumulates in the joints.

There are a number of causes for this condition, including deficiencies in bone-protecting vitamins such as calcium, vitamin C, vitamin D and magnesium.

The calcium in plant-based foods is more easily absorbed than that in milk. Foods that contain high levels of absorbable calcium include rhubarb, spinach, Chinese cabbage, tofu, kidney beans and pinto beans.

Rheumatoid Arthritis

Rheumatoid Arthritis (RA) is an autoimmune condition, which means your immune system sees harmless cells or tissues as harmful. In rheumatoid arthritis this leads to chronic inflammation in the joints.

Whilst supporting joint health is important, even more crucial is addressing the inflammation. You can do this simply and effectively by taking omega-3 (with a high EPA content – check the label and look for anything over 800 mg). Your next allies are probiotics. Not only will they support your digestive health, they will also encourage regulatory T-cell formation, which means more cells for your body to naturally fight inflammation. Probiotics can also help address your immune system's mixed-up response to normal tissues and cells.

Having rheumatoid arthritis puts you at a slightly higher risk of getting cancer of the lymph glands (lymphoma) so it's important to look after your spleen and lymphatic system (see the sections on the spleen on page 18 and on the lymphatic system on page 134).

If you've been experiencing all the symptoms of RA, but your blood test results are not confirming it, it's possible that you have seronegative RA. In most cases of rheumatoid arthritis, the individual tests positive for rheumatoid factor (RF) and/or anti-citrullinated peptide (CPP) antibodies. However, being seronegative, these markers will not show up in your test due to a lack of these specific antibodies in your blood.

Natural remedies include:

- **Avoiding the nightshade family (including tomatoes, potatoes, sweet peppers/capsicums, aubergines/eggplants, chillies and paprika) when you are experiencing a flare-up. They are known to exacerbate this condition**

- **Limiting intake of gluten and dairy**
- **Taking anti-inflammatory probiotics containing *Bifidobacterium infantis (B. infantis)* and *Saccharomyces boulardii (S. boulardii)***
- **Taking an omega-3 with high (at least 650 mg) EPA content.**

Food for bones include:

- **Nuts and seeds such as almonds and pecans**
- **Yoghurt**
- **Dairy products**
- **Sardines, salmon, tuna**
- **Eggs**
- **Spinach**
- **Fortified cereals.**

Gout

Gout is a form of arthritis that occurs when sharp crystals of uric acid collect between the joints causing painful inflammation. Uric acid is a chemical that the kidneys filter out of the blood through the urine.

Uric acid exists naturally in the body but is increased by high protein foods and foods containing a lot of a particular chemical called *purine*. The kidneys normally break down purines into uric acid and then eliminate it from the body. Foods high in purines are therefore best avoided.

People typically get gout because either their body produces too much uric acid or because their kidneys are not eliminating it effectively.

Foods to include	Foods to avoid
Berries	Alcohol
Bananas	Dairy
Celery	Anchovies
Cabbage	Mackerel
Parsley	Sardines
Kale	Peanuts
Rice	Most meats (even white)
Millet	Cauliflower
Corn/cornbread	Eggs (can eat in moderation)
Tofu/soy	Spinach (can eat in moderation)
Fish such as gurnard, snapper, cod, etc.	Marmite/vegemite
Cucumbers	Tomatoes (although they are low in purines, their high acidity aggravates gout)

Drinking herbal teas to support the kidneys is also helpful – there are many kidney cleansing teas on the market.

Other helpful drinks are:

- Apple cider vinegar – 2 tsp in a glass of warm water
- Dandelion or nettle tea
- Tart cherry juice
- Cucumber tea (use the peel of a third of a cucumber, add hot water, allow to infuse for 5 minutes then drink).

Supplements that can help are:

- Vitamin B5 *(vitamin B3 should be avoided)*
- Vitamin E
- Celery
- Turmeric (or curcumin)
- Boswelia.

Chapter 6

Blood and Circulatory Disorders

Earlier, on pages 34–36, I spoke of the signs and signals of nutrient deficiency. One example was a lack of magnesium, which can cause migraines, constipation and muscle cramps. Ignore these early warnings at your peril! Every muscle of your body needs magnesium to function properly and there is no more precious muscle than your heart. Eating foods rich in magnesium, together with essential fatty acids, fibre and co-enzyme Q10 will boost your heart health and lower the risk of disease or strokes.

Cholesterol Levels

Cholesterol is a waxy substance carried through your bloodstream attached to proteins called lipoproteins. It has several important functions, including making the outer coating of cells, contributing to the bile acids that digest food in your intestines and allowing your body to make Vitamin D and hormones like oestrogen in women and testosterone in men (in fact healthy cholesterol balance can support prostate health).

Many people are told their cholesterol is 'high' and agree to take medication for it. Incredibly, very few question what 'high' means. There are many natural ways that you can lower your cholesterol, but it's helpful to know what area to address. High cholesterol is usually caused by too much LDL/bad cholesterol, but there are other reasons too. Get to know your results.

Laboratories report in different formats depending on location and country (so I am not providing an example here to avoid confusion) but your doctor or health care provider can talk you through them in detail. Generally your cholesterol level is measured in units called millimoles per litre of blood, often shortened to mmol/L. Healthy adults should have a total cholesterol level below 5 mmol/L

Your results will include:

Total cholesterol level	The overall amount of cholesterol in your blood (the good and the bad)
Triglyceride level	A type of fat (lipid) in your blood
HDL (high density lipoproteins) level	The good guys (help clear fatty deposits from your arteries). The higher this number, the better
LDL (low density lipoproteins) level	The bad guys (can build up in your artery walls). The lower this number the better
Ratio	Total cholesterol level divided by HDL level

In 2020 research indicated we also need to consider other parts of 'bad' cholesterol, known as IDL, VLDL and lipoprotein(a). You may see these indicators featuring in your results.

There is undeniable evidence that diet has a positive effect on cholesterol management. A rewarding part of my job is to help clients stop taking their medication for cholesterol (if they choose to!)

Blood Pressure

Blood 'pressure' is the strength with which your blood pushes against your arteries as it pumps around your body. It is measured in millimetres of mercury (mmHg) and is shown in two separate numbers:

- **Systolic pressure – the pressure when your heart pushes blood out (the highest number in a reading)**
- **Diastolic pressure – the pressure when your heart rests between beats (the lowest number in a reading).**

A normal blood pressure is considered '120 over 80' (or 120/80 mmH) meaning a systolic pressure of 120 mmHg and a diastolic pressure of 80 mmHg. However, there are many reasons why your blood pressure may be higher or lower than this on any given day, so it's beneficial to have regular readings to get a true reflection.

My Mum was prescribed medication for high blood pressure in a one-off appointment with her doctor. She didn't need it. When I took her blood pressure a few months later, it was incredibly low and the medication was ditched immediately.

I'm always encouraging folk to 'know your numbers', and you need to know what your blood pressure is, alongside your cholesterol and blood sugars. We are all individuals and our bodies don't all fall into neat parameters. Interestingly, we are using the same parameters now as when blood pressure was first measured in the 1800s, begging the question if a review and update is warranted.

Currently:

- Normal blood pressure is considered to be between 90/60 mmHg and 120/80 mmHg
- High blood pressure is considered to be 140/90 mmHg or higher
- Low blood pressure is considered to be 90/60 mmHg or lower.

High Blood Pressure (Hypertension)

As noted above, your blood pressure will be considered high if it is consistently over 140/90. Causes include being overweight, having too much salt in your diet, drinking too much alcohol, suffering from stress, not getting enough exercise and having food intolerances (the latter very rarely considered). Symptoms can include fatigue and headaches It's sadly all too easy to take a medication to treat the symptom of high blood pressure rather than to investigate and address the cause(s), but as all medications come with side effects, it's always better to see if you can naturally reduce your blood pressure.

Natural Remedies Include:

- Grapes
- Bananas
- Ginger
- Garlic
- Onions
- Test food intolerances
- Exercise
- Mindfulness.

Low Blood Pressure (Hypotension)

I have had low blood pressure all my life and it's never been an issue for me. However for some it is a concern, with symptoms including dizzy spells, fainting, blurred vision and heart palpitations, as reduced blood pressure restricts the amount of blood flowing to the brain and other organs. Low cortisol is another potential cause.

Natural Remedies Include:

- Licorice root
- Beetroot
- Drink more water
- Take B12 and folate supplements.

Heart Attack (Myocardial Infarction)

So now we know what blood pressure is (and the importance of becoming familiar with our own), what happens when blood flow to the muscles of your heart is restricted? If your heart is denied blood, it won't be able to function ... and neither will you!

If blood flow is compromised, you may experience pain in the left side or centre of your chest, which can spread into your shoulder, arm, back, neck or jaw. These symptoms may be subtle at first, unlike the chest clenching, gasping dramatics portrayed on film, but they shouldn't be ignored. If blood flow stops altogether, it leads to a sudden cardiac arrest, where the heart stops beating.

Keeping your arteries clear is crucial, as is improving your circulation by eating the following foods:

- Beans
- Beetroot
- Berries
- Broccoli
- Cinnamon
- Flax seeds
- Garlic
- Ginger
- Lemons
- Limes
- Oats
- Oily fish
- Onions.

Angina

This condition (not a disease) occurs when blood flow to the heart is restricted.

There are two types of angina: stable angina is the most common and is often triggered by exercise and/or stress. Symptoms quickly disappear within a few moments of resting and calming the body. Unstable angina is less common and doesn't appear to have specific triggers. Attacks are unpredictable and do not always disappear after resting.

Natural remedies include:

- Apple cider vinegar
- Garlic
- Onions
- Turmeric
- Ginger
- Olive Oil
- Co-enzyme Q10 supplement.

Atrial Fibrillation

This condition causes an irregular heartbeat and increases the risk of having a stroke. Symptoms are diverse but signs to look for would be heart palpitations, shortness of breath, light-headedness, confusion and, sometimes, chest pain.

Healthy food choices include:

- Leafy greens
- Oily fish
- Nuts and seeds – flax seeds, chia seeds
- Whole grains
- Berries
- Avocados.

Meanwhile, avoid:

- Drinking excessive amounts of alcohol, particularly binge drinking
- Being overweight (see Appendix 1, page 190 for Tips for Weight Loss)
- Drinking lots of caffeine, such as tea, coffee or energy drinks
- Taking illegal drugs, particularly amphetamines or cocaine
- Smoking.

Stroke

Although mostly affecting older people, anyone can have a stroke, including children. Those with diabetes and/or high blood pressure are at greater risk. This serious life-threatening condition occurs when the blood supply to part of the brain is cut off. There is a useful and memorable check for the main symptoms using the word FAST:

- Face – the face may have dropped on one side, the person may not be able to smile, or their mouth or eye may have drooped.
- Arms – the person may not be able to lift both arms and keep them there because of weakness or numbness in one arm.
- Speech – their speech may be slurred or garbled, or the person may not be able to talk at all despite appearing to be awake; they may also have problems understanding what you're saying to them.
- Time – dial for an ambulance immediately if you notice any of these signs or symptoms.

However, there are other signs to watch out for too including blurred vision, severe headache, confusion and dizziness.

Research has indicated that a Mediterranean diet rich in antioxidants, vitamins, potassium, calcium, vegetables, fruits, whole grains and oily fish can lower the risk of having a stroke. Unsurprisingly , these foods can also aid in recovery.

Varicose Veins

Veins help pump blood towards the heart. Veins in the leg have to move the blood upwards, and so they have valves in them to help prevent the blood flowing backwards. If the veins are faulty, blood starts to collect in little pools rather than flowing up to the heart. This causes the vein to stretch and bulge.

Natural remedies include:

- Any foods that support circulation are therefore helpful e.g. blueberries, grapes, dark chocolate (I know!), pumpkin seeds and leafy greens
- Foods rich in vitamin C will strengthen the walls of the veins, promoting healing and protecting membranes against damaging free-radicals.

Supplements:

- Co-enzyme Q10
- Garlic
- Vitamin C
- Vitamin E.

Chapter 7
Lung Disorders

Asthma

Asthma can affect anyone at any age and ranges from mild, barely noticeable symptoms to life-threatening. Airways narrow and swell and extra mucus is produced, making breathing difficult, leading to wheeziness and shortness of breath. It is often accompanied by a cough. Natural cures are the same for those listed below for COPD.

Chronic Obstructive Pulmonary Disease (COPD)

This is a condition affecting the lungs and where breathing is difficult. COPD is a general term for progressive respiratory diseases like emphysema and chronic bronchitis. Airflow gradually decreases over time and tissues in the airway become increasingly inflamed.

Symptoms include:

- Shortness of breath
- Chest pain
- Blue tinted skin (cyanosis)
- Swelling of the feet
- Coughing
- Repeated lung infections
- A 'barrel' chest
- Excess phlegm
- Fatigue
- Mood or memory problems
- Wheezing
- Fever
- Unexplained weight loss.

Studies have shown that preservatives (especially sulphur dioxide, no. 220) are responsible for triggering certain respiratory conditions, so it's important to have as much fresh food as possible. Reducing or even eliminating foods with preservatives will also reduce the presence of harmful yeasts in your system.

Natural remedies include:

- Vitamins A, C and E
- Vitamin D
- Magnesium
- Zinc
- Peppermint tea
- Thyme
- Eucalyptus oil.

Chapter 8
Pregnancy

Pregnancy is not a disease, but is important to eat well to make sure you and your baby stay as healthy as possible.

Research has indicated that choline assists the brain development of foetuses, so it's important that you get a good intake of choline-rich foods such as eggs, beef, cauliflower, almonds and tofu. Aim for 3.5 g (3500 mg) per day. (Above this, adverse effects can include low blood pressure, diarrhoea and a fishy body odour – not pleasant!)

Eating a diet rich in fruits and vegetables, whole grains, legumes and nuts and consuming a low to moderate amount of dairy products, eggs and red meat will help protect your baby from allergies, eczema and asthma during childhood. This Mediterranean-type diet is high in fibre, antioxidants, monounsaturated fatty acids and omega-3 fatty acids, and is low in saturated fats.

Avoid licorice; it contains glycyrrhizin. Prenatal exposure to glyrrhizin is connected with preterm birth and detrimental effects on cognitive performance during childhood.

During your pregnancy, limit your intake of caffeine and make sure any meat you have is thoroughly cooked because of the risk of contamination with coliform bacteria, listeria, toxoplasmosis and salmonella.

Also avoid:

- Unpasteurised milk
- Soft cheeses such as brie and camembert
- Raw or undercooked eggs
- Patés
- Liver and liver products
- Ready-to-eat salads from the delicatessen counters at the supermarket.

Chapter 9

Immune System Disorders

The Lymphatic System

Lymph is a clear substance that passes just under the surface of your skin via vessels, nodes and glands throughout your body. The flow slows down as it passes through the ear canal and sinus area. If spleen action is weak, the movement of lymph slows down even more and can cause headaches, 'blocked' sinuses, itchy ears, swollen glands and even 'waxy' ears.

Your body produces ear wax to defend your ears against infection. It is produced by glands in the outer ear canal, which are part of your lymphatic system. If you are uncomfortably aware of its presence, this may indicate that your lymphatic flow is impaired due to the inefficiency of your spleen. Ear wax can become thicker if too much saturated fat is in your diet, so be sure to reduce your intake of fatty foods, especially while your spleen action is weak. If your problem isn't too bad, then simply using a couple of drops of olive oil in each ear once or twice a week should help.

Your tonsils and appendix are also part of your lymphatic system. If you've had either of these removed, you would do well to cheer up your spleen! Eat foods such as beetroot, parsnips, cucumber, barley and fennel to support your spleen and lymphatic system, consider a lymphatic drainage massage, and try dry skin brushing to stimulate and improve lymphatic flow.

Hay Fever

Whilst most of us welcome the Spring season, as many as 40% will be dreading the all too familiar itchy eyes, stuffy nose, sneezing and fatigue – and the many other symptoms that hay fever (allergic rhinitis) brings at this time of year.

The reason why some people are more prone than others is all down to individual immune response. When certain allergens such as pollens enter the body, vulnerable immune systems see them as invaders and release the chemical histamine to destroy them. It's the production and circulation of histamine in the system that causes the adverse side effects that sufferers know all too well. However, there is much that can be done to alleviate, if not control histamine production. Whilst medications can bring almost as many unwanted side effects (e.g. drowsiness, dry mouth, headaches, etc.), there are plenty of natural antihistamines in our foods.

The good guys:

- Vitamin C – oranges, lemons, mandarins, capsicums, broccoli, cauliflower
- Quercetin (a phytochemical) – apples, apricots, red onions, red grapes, berries
- Spirulina – these algae have proven anti-histamine effects
- Probiotics – more evidence is emerging that probiotics (healthy bacteria) can help combat the effects of grass and tree pollen in particular. Look for products that contain *Paracasei*.

The bad guys:

- Whilst foods can help alleviate symptoms, it's worth knowing that some foods can make things worse. For instance, carrot family vegetables contain specific molecules called psoralens that can exacerbate hay fever symptoms in some people. Notice if your symptoms worsen after you eat carrots, celery, turnips, parsley, etc. Unidentified food intolerances will also worsen hay fever symptoms.

Autoimmune diseases

This one resonates with me, because I have one! An autoimmune disease arises when your immune system strikes out against healthy cells, harming your tissues and causing loss of normal bodily functioning. This can happen anywhere in your body and that's why there are so many autoimmune conditions.

It's never been known why the body decides to attack itself in this way – but I have a theory. Every single person I have ever seen with an autoimmune condition of any type has also had food intolerances. My theory is this: the food we eat should be nourishing our cells. When food enters our mouths, our systems gear up to process it and send the nutrients where they need to go. If we are intolerant to that food, however, our systems see it as an invader and react the same as they would to any other invader (e.g. pet hair, pollen, a virus) by releasing antibodies to fight back. The confusion arises due to the fact that one minute we are telling our bodies that nutrients are on their way to feed our cells, the next thing we have sent in 'the enemy'! No wonder our poor defences get mixed up! My belief is that this then impacts on other systems that are trying to work efficiently, but we have created internal chaos!

The body makes different immunoglobulins to combat different antigens. For example, the antibody for chickenpox isn't the same as the antibody for mononucleosis. Sometimes, the body may even mistakenly make antibodies against itself, treating healthy organs and tissues like foreign invaders. This is called an autoimmune disease.

The five subclasses of antibodies are:

- **Immunoglobulin A (IgA)**, which is found in high concentrations in the mucous membranes, particularly those lining the respiratory passages and gastrointestinal tract, as well as in saliva and tears
- **Immunoglobulin G (IgG)**, the most abundant type of antibody, is found in all body fluids and protects against bacterial and viral infections

- **Immunoglobulin M (IgM)**, which is found mainly in the blood and lymph fluid, is the first antibody to be made by the body to fight a new infection

- **Immunoglobulin E (IgE)**, which is associated mainly with allergic reactions (when the immune system overreacts to environmental antigens such as pollen or pet dander), is found in the lungs, skin and mucous membranes

- **Immunoglobulin D (IgD)**, which exists in small amounts in the blood, is the least understood antibody.

IgA, IgG and IgM are often measured together. That way, they can give doctors important information about immune system functioning, especially relating to infection or autoimmune disease.

Once an antibody is produced against a specific antigen, the next time that antigen enters the body, the immune system 'remembers' its response and produces more of the same antibodies. In that way, checking for the presence of specific immunoglobulins in the blood can be helpful in diagnosing or ruling out infections or certain other illnesses.

Doctors also rely on the immunoglobulin test as one of the tools to help diagnose immunodeficiencies (when the immune system isn't working properly). A person can be born with an immunodeficiency or acquire it through infection, disease, malnutrition, burns, or as a side effect of medicines. Doctors may suspect an immunodeficiency in a child who experiences frequent or unusual infections.

Immunoglobulin levels are also used as part of an evaluation for autoimmune conditions such as juvenile idiopathic arthritis, lupus, and celiac disease.

There are scores of identified autoimmune conditions ranging from mild to severe, and they include:

- IBD (inflammatory bowel disease, including Crohn's disease and ulcerative colitis)
- Rheumatoid arthritis
- Raynaud's disease
- Type 1 diabetes
- Multiple sclerosis
- Systemic lupus erythematosus (Lupus)
- Scleroderma (thickening and hardening of the skin)
- Sjogren's syndrome (chronic dryness of the body, eyes, mouth, vagina, etc.)
- Graves' disease (overproduction of thyroid hormones)
- Hashimoto's disease (underproduction of thyroid hormones)
- Glomerulonephritis (kidney inflammation that can lead to kidney failure)
- Guillain-Barre' syndrome (weakness, numbness and paralysis)
- Psoriasis (inflammatory skin disease)

It is possible to have more than one autoimmune disease. After all, if the body is indeed confused, then defences are lower and unable to fight back or establish friend from foe.

Autoimmune diseases don't always have a clear pattern of symptoms, so they can be difficult to diagnose. It's easy to assume that many symptoms are all part and parcel of ageing. I saw a 74-year-old lady once who went to her doctor complaining that she wasn't herself. She told him she couldn't quite put her finger on it, but she knew she "wasn't right". She described various, what appeared to be innocuous-sounding symptoms, and he told her not to worry and that she was simply "getting old". Fortunately, she wasn't satisfied with that answer and sought advice elsewhere and came to one of my clinics. I ran some tests, including one that looks for autoimmune conditions (I had a hunch after I'd heard her collective symptoms), and they revealed that she had lupus. Over the years, I have picked up many cases of autoimmune disease where other clients were similarly dismissed.

Whilst there are no clear symptoms for autoimmune diseases, one thing they **all** have in common is chronic inflammation, and I have found that controlling the inflammation **naturally** is key to managing symptoms. I underline the word naturally because the last thing we want to do to a mixed up, confused system that doesn't know a friend from a foe, is to bombard it with aggressive painkillers and anti-inflammatory drugs! Happily, there are a number of less villainous options to choose from. Omega-3 essential fatty acids, eicosapentaenoic acid (EPA) and docosahexaenoic acid (DHA) have natural anti-inflammatory and painkilling properties and can be a powerful ally.

The omega-3 from fish is not the same as the omega-3 from fruits and vegetables. Although wonderful essential fatty acids, they do not contain EPA and DHA. I'm often asked about vegan fish oil alternatives. Algae is the only plant-based source of EPA and DHA omega-3 and some companies produce a vegan fish oil supplement based on that. However, the levels are not as high as a pure fish oil supplement.

Oily fish like salmon, tuna and mackerel are rich in EPA and DHA, but most average diets don't contain enough to control the inflammation of an autoimmune condition and supplementing can be hugely beneficial. Look for a brand that offers at least 800 mg of each (it will be listed on the label).

Turmeric is a powerful, yet mild-tasting spice that also offers great pain-killing and anti-inflammatory properties. Curcumin, its derivative, is also highly recommended.

Last, but certainly not least, we return to our wonderful friends, probiotics. Unlike dangerous drugs, probiotics (especially those containing the *Lactobacillus plantarum* and/or *Streptococcus salivarius* varieties) can help address the immune system's mixed-up response to normal tissues and cells. Indeed, emerging research is linking insufficient gut bacteria to autoimmune conditions and gut permeability. Watch this space!

Avoiding nightshades

The nightshade family of foods are known to trigger inflammatory responses in systems that are vulnerable, and for that reason they are best avoided when you have an autoimmune condition, especially during flare-ups. They've been mentioned before but it doesn't hurt to be reminded. They include:

- **Tomatoes – regardless of whether they are raw or cooked**
- **Potatoes – including all potato products, such as crisps**
- **Capsicums/sweet peppers**
- **Aubergines/eggplant**
- **Chillies.**

There are others, but these are the most commonly used foods. You do not (should not) need to exclude them permanently.

Finally, whilst it seems that there is no support for autoimmune conditions, in my own personal and clinical experience, take heart that you can certainly live in long-term remission, as if you don't have it at all. Of course, the type and extent of the condition will obviously play a part in individual cases, together with any other health issues, but you can take back some control by using food as medicine and healing your gut.

Chapter 10

Chronic Fatigue Syndrome

For a long time, Chronic Fatigue Syndrome (CFS) was not recognised by doctors. In 2015, the National Academy of Medicine in America (formerly known as the Institute of Medicine) filed a report with the government calling for better diagnosis and acceptance of the condition, even suggesting a name change to Systemic Exertion Intolerance Disease (SEID).

Whatever its name, I can certainly confirm that this is a very real and challenging health issue. Sadly, many clients I see with this condition feel isolated from their friends and family, who believe the doctor's conclusion that it's all in their head. The collection of seemingly unrelated (yet often utterly debilitating) symptoms makes diagnosis difficult. It takes time and effort through the right questioning and testing to help identify what the body needs. One of the most fundamental revelations I discovered from the thousands of clients I've seen is that the majority (if not all) had unidentified food intolerances. **I would strongly urge you to have a food intolerance test if you feel you have any of the CFS-related conditions.** As I've said before, it's not always gluten and dairy.

The following conditions sit under the CFS umbrella.

Fibromyalgia

Fibromyalgia affects the muscles and soft tissues in the body. I once had a client who couldn't even tolerate the pressure of a gentle shower. Accompanied with fatigue and low moods, this condition can really take a toll – if it's allowed to! Early diagnosis and natural therapies can very quickly return the body to a state of ongoing remission. Believe me, I have witnessed the most extreme transformations from people who were suffering, including the lady mentioned earlier. There is always something you can do!

I find that sufferers typically have low levels of cortisol. Among other symptoms, low cortisol secretion is linked to low energy, muscle weakness and pain, thyroid dysfunction, depression, low immunity and sleep disorders.

Myalgic Encephalomyelitis (ME)

This illness affects the neurological, immune, musculoskeletal, endocrine and cardiovascular systems. Symptoms are diverse and varied and affect sufferers in different ways. Although there may be some generic 'treatments', every case has to be looked at in its own merit. A crucial common link for everyone, however, appears to be depletion of magnesium stores in the body. I find that increasing magnesium levels in my clients' diets has a major impact on their health and energy. This is largely due to the fact that magnesium helps ATP (Adenosine Triphosphate) synthesis. ATP naturally occurs in the body and, amongst its many functions, it prevents fatigue, increases stamina, supports muscular strength and stability and supports the mitochondria (our cell's power sources!).

For CFS, ME and fibromyalgia, natural remedies include:

- A probiotic containing *Saccharomyces boulardii*
- Magnesium (levels are often extremely low in sufferers of these conditions)
- Co-enzyme Q10 (300 mg if considering a supplement)
- Omega-3 (oily fish or supplement containing EPA of over 500 mg)
- Zinc (40 mg if considering a supplement. Make sure it contains copper too).

Adrenal Fatigue

Your adrenals are walnut-shaped glands that sit just above your kidneys. Your body is designed to release two hormones, adrenalin and cortisol, to help you cope with stressful situations and then rest in between. This is part of our innate human response to attack or danger of any kind, known as our fight or flight response.

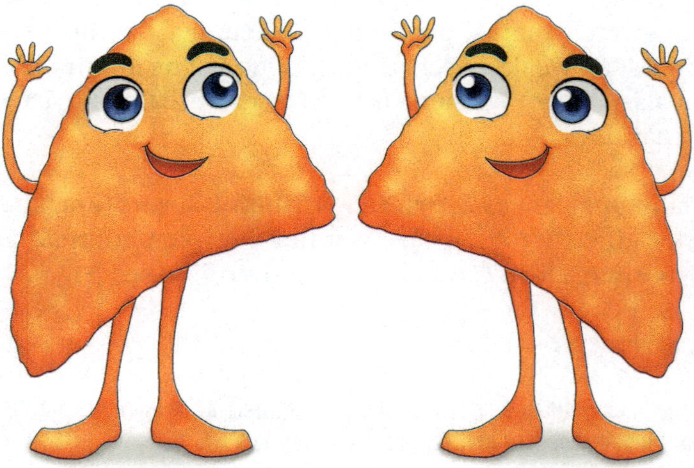

In today's busy life, our adrenals are working far harder than nature ever intended. Many of us are juggling work, children, caring for parents, finances, relationships and more. Not much chance of resting then! The more stress we are subjected to, the more the stress hormones are released. This causes the release of glucose, because in a true fight-or-flight state, we would need that glucose for energy to run or fight. But today's stresses are not the life-threatening challenges we once faced and the glucose can lead to increased blood sugar levels, contributing to weight gain, lethargy and dizzy spells. Sleep can also be affected as you are never switching your engine off. Apart from the stress hormones, the adrenals also produce a natural steroid hormone. If you are taking prednisone medication for an extended period of time, it will cause your adrenal glands to reduce cortisol production. Amongst other symptoms, low cortisol can cause extreme fatigue, weight loss, digestive issues and low blood pressure. Addison's disease (also known as adrenal insufficiency) is a condition that can develop if low cortisol production persists.

Prolonged exposure to cortisol may lead to a condition known as Cushing's syndrome. Signs and symptoms may include high blood pressure, abdominal obesity but with thin arms and legs, reddish stretch marks, a round red face, a fat lump between the shoulders, weak muscles, weak bones, acne and fragile skin that heals poorly. Women may have more hair and irregular menstruation.

Adrenalin imbalances interfere with iodine absorption, and that can affect the thyroid. There is a link between adrenal fatigue and hypothyroidism (an underactive thyroid – see page 79).

Natural remedies include:

- Breathing techniques such as Buteyko can help calm your system, lower your blood pressure and support your adrenals
- Eat plenty of colourful fruits and vegetables and oily fish
- Eat dark chocolate to lift your mood and raise serotonin levels
- Identify and eliminate any foods you are intolerant to.

Long Covid

Long Covid is the effects of Covid-19 that continue for weeks or months beyond the initial illness. At the time of writing, early statistics are showing that those most affected are in the 40–55-year-old age bracket.

Symptoms are many and varied and include fatigue, headaches, loss of smell and taste, shortness of breath, persistent cough, joint pain, sore throat, digestive issues and weight fluctuations.

Whilst this is still a relatively new condition, already it's clear that diet and supplements can play a role in addressing and easing the symptoms associated with it.

It appears that plant-based and/or fish diets reduce the severity of symptoms in those contracting Covid-19, and ease the symptoms of those then who go on to experience long Covid *(Seidelman et al, June 2021)*. This is due to the positive effect these foods have on the immune system, and also the anti-inflammatory properties they possess.

I was particularly pleased when I read a report linking probiotic use to better outcomes for Long Covid patients. Led by experts from Addenbrooke's Hospital in Cambridge, the University of Bedfordshire and Bedfordshire Hospitals NHS Foundation Trust, the research revealed that coughs, fatigue, gut issues and overall well-being all improved for those taking probiotics compared to those who didn't. I've certainly been telling all my clients to have probiotics to boost their immune system ever since covid struck.

Natural remedies include:

- Staying hydrated if appetite loss is a symptom (have an electrolyte drink, or consider a fortified liquid supplement)
- Probiotics (and fermented food). The species *Saccharomyces boulardii* is especially helpful
- Ginseng
- Echinacea
- Vitamin C
- Vitamin D
- Zinc.

Chapter 11
Cancer

If there's a condition that strikes fear into most people more than any other, it's cancer. It seems to strike anyone, anywhere, at any time, with seemingly no catalyst. So let's take a closer look at what's happening and what we can do about it.

In *very* simple terms a normal, healthy cell goes through a lifecycle – rather like us. It is 'born', it does its job in our body throughout its lifespan and, when it reaches a certain stage of maturity, it says, "I've done a very good job here, I'm off" (well, it would do if cells could speak!). Then it kills itself (a stage known as apoptosis), which triggers the release of another cell. This new cell replicates what the previous cell has done, although like any copy, it doesn't do quite as good a job, and that's how we age. Fabulous!

However, some cells get to the apoptosis stage and don't kill themselves, instead they linger on and start to mutate. The mutations develop into an uncontrolled growth – a cluster of mutated cells. At this point, you would feel a lump. The good news is that at this stage, the lump is benign (not cancerous). What causes it to become cancerous is when it comes into contact with free radicals. These are the usual suspects: pollution, food additives, tobacco smoke, pesticides, etc. If the free radicals meet the benign tumour and oxidise on contact, the tumour now becomes cancerous. It is the oxidisation of the free radicals that leads to a cancerous tumour ... which is why your **anti**oxidants are so important.

So why should someone be more prone to having misbehaving cells than anyone else? Well, it's all about risk factors, and it helps to know what yours are.

- **Hereditary:** is there's a prevalence of cancer, especially a particular type, in your family?
- **Environmental:** are you living in a city where there is high lead pollution? Perhaps you live close to a telegraph pole? Maybe you're near an orchard or farmland where sprays and pesticides are used?
- **Hormones:** early menstruation (before 12 years old), and the use of hormone replacement therapy and the birth control pill have been linked with an increased risk of female cancers, including breast and ovarian.
- **Exposure to toxins:** make-up, deodorant, plastic drinking bottles (they contain a chemical called bisphenol-A – look for BPA-free bottles) and mobile phones all contribute to toxin levels.
- **Soil depletion:** zinc and selenium are two nutrients that help fight cancer. New Zealand soils, for example, are depleted in these.
- **Poor digestive health:** this results in malabsorption of cancer-fighting antioxidants.
- **Diet:** this may be nutrient-deficient or too acidic (see below).
- **Processed foods:** these are high in colourings, food additives and preservatives.
- **Insufficient healthy bacteria:** oh yes, our little probiotic friends appear again as an ally.
- **Stress, anger and 'holding on' to bad memories and traumas:** stress creates many imbalances in the system and increases acidity. We can't control the curve balls that life throws us, but we can equip our system to deal with the fall-out.

Natural remedies include:

- Apple cider vinegar. This will alkalise your system and aid digestion. Tumours thrive in an acidic environment but do not survive in an alkaline one
- Cut back on added sugars. Sugar creates many imbalances in the system and raises acidity. No more than 30 g of sugar a day (no more than 5 g per serving)

- A glass of vegetable juice a day will help fight free radicals. Always include broccoli florets – broccoli has been proven to help cancer cells 'commit suicide'!
- Ginger, turmeric and carrots together have been shown to have the same impact on destroying cancerous cells as chemotherapy.

Useful supplements to help fight cancerous cells include:

- Selenium (good food source - try two Brazil nuts per day)
- Co-enzyme Q10 (good food source - broccoli)
- Zinc (good food sources - fish, pumpkin seeds and dark green veg)
- Vitamin C (good food sources berries, watercress).

Part 3

Medications, Supplements and Eating Well

Remembering that the human body is just a series of cells (trillions of them!) all waiting for nutrients, it's easy to see why we need a good, all-round diet packed with variety and colour to provide all the nutrients our cells need to function.

We've acknowledged that there are many barriers to nutrients reaching the cells – stress, toxins, food intolerances and poor digestive health. This leads to health issues that we look to resolve. Hopefully you'll be more inclined to look for natural remedies if you've read this far, but if medications are part of your choices then do please get to know as much as you can about them, especially if you're having repeat prescriptions.

Chapter 1

Medication and Food Conflicts

I hope that I am not sending out the message that all medication is evil and we shouldn't have it. On the contrary, I think we are lucky to be living in an age where science has progressed so much that we are in a position to be able to tackle some stubborn diseases and viruses with potent drugs.

But (you knew the 'but' was coming didn't you!), just as food affects everyone differently, so does medication. What works for one person may not work for another. Beyond that, my message is about raising awareness of the choices you have. Medication is certainly one of them, but if you don't know about other remedies and natural supports, how can you make the best choice for yourself?

Ever since I started in practice, I have been underlining the importance of checking the side effects of medications to individual clients. In my speaking engagements I am pleased to emphasise this message to a wider audience. (After one such talk, a man contacted me later to say, "I think you have literally saved my life! I saw my doctor after your talk, and I have been taken off three medications that were causing me mental issues, and I hadn't made the link".)

It frustrates me that there are reports of the increase in conditions like Alzheimer's , dementia and Parkinsonism, and yet when we look at the side effects of medications, very many (too many) reveal that long-term use can cause these conditions. It's the same with depression and anxiety. The list below shows some common medications used for common medical conditions and the potential side effects that they can have.

Condition	Medication	Side Effects
Asthma	Prednisone	Severe depression, personality changes, extreme sadness
Underactive thyroid	Levothyroxine	Anxiety, depression, sleep disruption
Diabetes	Metformin	Panic attacks, anxiety, depression
High cholesterol	Atorvastatin, Simvastatin	Nightmares, nervousness, depression

What if you were a person with high cholesterol, an underactive thyroid and high blood pressure taking medications to treat all three? You might well be another dementia statistic in years to come.

After my many years in practice, I can almost predict what medication people are taking. As they go through their ailments, I know down to the brand name the medication they are about to tell me they have been prescribed. Let's take blood pressure. Eight people with high blood pressure are all taking benazepril. Well, isn't that interesting, when you consider that these people include:

- A highly-stressed businesswoman
- A man going through a bitter divorce
- An older lady with an undiscovered food intolerance

- A mid-40s man who is reacting to a different medication for his high cholesterol
- A lady who rarely exercises as she has painful osteoarthritis
- An anxious 30-year-old
- An overweight man in his 60s
- A menopausal lady who can't sleep.

All completely different people with completely different causes for their high blood pressure – and yet all on exactly the same medication to control it. *Treating the symptom but not addressing the cause!* In all of these cases, if the time was taken to establish what lay behind the symptom of the high blood pressure, the cause would be revealed, and addressed.

Amongst the worst offenders for side effects are the statin drugs, used to lower cholesterol. Again, we are not looking at why the individual has high cholesterol in the first place. Is it hereditary? Is it due to poor diet? Is it through lack of exercise? And what aspect of the cholesterol needs to be targeted?

If you are taking statin drugs, they will bring down your LDL cholesterol. Of course they will, that's what they are designed to do. Marvellous! Your cholesterol is now in the nice safe 'bracket of normal' where we want you to be. But have you ever thought how the statin achieved such greatness? It has done its job by leeching onto your cells and, if that cell was carrying bad cholesterol, the statin drug will take it away. Excellent, well done statin. Oh, but what's happening now? The statin drug has leeched onto a cell that was carrying magnesium for your muscles and now you are experiencing cramps and headaches. Never mind, look at your lovely cholesterol reading! What's that? The statin has leeched a cell carrying calcium to your bones, and now you are having joint pain and fatigue. Well cheer up, your cholesterol's perfect. Whoops, the statin has interfered with your zinc supply and now you are forgetting everything. Oh dear, well let's hope you remember how great your cholesterol is!

My Mum's Story

Whilst I was in New Zealand preaching to the world and his wife about the dangerous side effects of medications, my own mother was falling victim to just that on the other side of the world.

It transpired that, following a health check on her 83rd birthday, she was prescribed a raft of medication for everything from high blood pressure to an overactive bladder, despite the fact that she suffered with neither. I wasn't aware of this until it was too late.

Mum had always been fit, happy and healthy, and often taken for 20 years younger. Sharp minded with a great sense of humour, she loved life and took pleasure in regularly traveling with my dad to see her grandchildren.

I had noticed that on my previous couple of visits home, Mum was very slow on her feet and didn't seem as confident as usual. She was also very weepy, which was upsetting to witness and so unlike her. Given that my visits were usually confined to Christmas they were short and frantic with a host of other family members, and I didn't really sit down and talk to Mum at length about her health.

The change in her prompted my decision to return to the UK, so that I could be with both her and Dad in their golden years. Within days of my return, Mum informed me that she had been diagnosed with Parkinson's disease. What?! She told me she had seen a geriatrician who had concluded her various collection of symptoms were the result of having Parkinson's disease and promptly prescribed the common medication for it. Whoa ... hold on.

I recall Mum saying she hadn't felt 'right' since her 83rd birthday. That got me thinking about her health check and the medications she was prescribed at that time. I asked her to tell me all her symptoms, and I made a list (which was worryingly long). I then looked at her medications and the side effects almost mirrored the list I had. Mum admitted that she was overwhelmed with everything she had to take.

One of the medications, Vesicare (prescribed for an overactive bladder) adversely affects the central nervous system. It shouldn't be given for a prolonged period of time, but my Mum had had a repeat prescription for a number of years. Parkinson's is a condition of the central nervous system.

I went with her to see her doctor and we discussed our concerns. He agreed that she could stop taking all the medications to see how her body responded. On our return 4 weeks later, her blood pressure was perfect (it always had been), she had no bladder issues (she'd never had any), she had stopped hallucinating and she was far more positive mentally. However, she still had impaired mobility and other symptoms of Parkinsonism.

There are a number of triggers for Parkinsonism including:

- **Parkinson's disease (impaired cells in the brain)**
- **The after-effects of a stroke (vascular Parkinsonism)**
- **Side effects of specific medications, a condition known as drug-induced Parkinsonism (DIP).**

My mum undoubtedly has DIP. That said, she also reported that she felt she had had "a slight stroke a while ago" which, although recorded by the geriatrician, had never been followed up. In most cases of DIP, once the medication is stopped, the negative symptoms stop. However, the longer an individual remains on the medication, the less likely they are to return to their normal state and, sadly, my mum had been on hers too long.

Meanwhile, Mum's kidney function was appalling, as evidenced in her blood test results. Nothing was being done about the situation because, as she was told, "it's wear and tear". Maybe, but that doesn't mean it can't be improved! After a few months of herbal remedies, my Mum's kidney function was better. Still not great, but at least things were improving.

During the pandemic lockdown, my mum injured her shin and it bled profusely. My dad called the doctor who sent someone along to tend the wound. A few days later, my mum's leg was swollen and there was an incredible loss of plasma fluid. Another doctor came to visit and prescribed furosemide (a medication used to control fluid levels in the body). However, furosemide shouldn't be given to someone with certain kidney issues, which my mum had. After starting on the medication, she became violently sick.

My parents didn't connect the sickness to the medication for the leg, so when my dad called the doctor and reported my mum's vomiting, another doctor was sent round to see her. Instead of realising it was the furosemide causing the sickness, the doctor decided to prescribe an anti-nausea medication called metoclopramide. METOCLOPRAMIDE SHOULD NOT BE GIVEN TO ANYONE WITH PARKINSON'S. Soon after taking this mediation, my mum ground to a halt. All of her Parkinson's symptoms became ten times worse. She couldn't stand, couldn't see, couldn't eat and was utterly confused.

I hadn't been able to visit my parents due to Covid restrictions, but I called the day after the metoclopramide had been prescribed. As soon as my Dad told me how bad my Mum was, I asked him to tell me the names of the medications she was on. AAAGGHHH! I told him she should stop them immediately whilst I tried to contact her doctor and Parkinson's specialist. Both agreed that a mistake had been made and apologised. My mum is still living with the side effects of this awful blunder, and it set her back after she was progressing so well.

To say I am frustrated by my Mum's situation is an understatement. Sadly, I know she is not alone. There are literally millions of people all over the world suffering from symptoms (Parkinsonism being just one) that have been caused by medications that they simply don't need; or, if they do, then the side effects are worse than the condition being treated. Statistics are proving that cases of dementia and Alzheimer's are on the rise. Before we throw yet more money into research, let's take a close look at the medications we are prescribing!

Please, please, please, if you or anyone you know is taking a medication of any sort for any reason, check the side effects. My message is not about ditching medications. As mentioned earlier, I recognise that we are privileged to be living in an age and time when research can offer so much. But just as food affects us all differently, so do medications. One man's meat is quite literally another man's poison.

Food and Medication

Another area for concern is the little-known, or certainly little publicised, fact that certain foods interfere with the effectiveness of some medications. Below are a few examples.

Levothyroxine/Synthroid

This medication is a man-made thyroid hormone used to treat hypothyroidism (an underactive thyroid). You should seek a blood test confirming your TSH (Thyroid Stimulating Hormone) and T4 (Thyroxine) levels before resorting to medication. Always ask to see a copy of your results and be sure to ask for regular tests – at least 6 monthly – to ensure your medication is still required.

Whilst taking this medication, you need to avoid foods that block the use of iodine, including:

- **Soy products (lecithin, tofu, etc.)**
- **Broccoli (especially raw)**
- **Brussel sprouts**
- **Cabbage (especially raw – e.g. coleslaw)**
- **Cauliflower (especially raw)**
- **Kale**
- **Millet**
- **Peaches**
- **Peanuts and pine nuts**
- **Radishes**
- **Spinach**
- **Strawberries**
- **Turnips.**

To help thyroid medication work more effectively, take it well away from any of the foods listed (at least two hours before or after) to ensure full absorption of the medication. At the same time, it will help if you increase your intake of iodine (easily absorbable from sea vegetables such as spirulina, dulse and kelp), selenium, folic acid and vitamin E.

If you take iron and calcium supplements with this medication, leave at least 4 hours between each. Steer clear of decongestants too.

High Blood Pressure Medications

These include drugs such as Losartan, Amlodipine, Lisinopril and Propranolol.

Avoid grapefruits and grapefruit juice. Limit your intake of potassium-rich foods (e.g. bananas, cantaloupe, grapefruits, oranges, tomato juice, prunes, honeydew melons, molasses and potatoes) and protein-rich foods (e.g. meat and dairy – Atkins and keto followers beware!).

Warfarin (an Anticoagulant)

Avoid vitamin K-rich foods (e.g. liver, broccoli, Brussel sprouts, cabbage, green leafy vegetables, asparagus, avocados, green tea, mayonnaise, olive oil, and soybean oil).

Metformin (for Type-2 Diabetes and Polycystic Ovary Syndrome)

Increase your intake of vitamin B12-rich foods (e.g. beef, pork, sardines, tuna, trout, salmon and fortified cereals).

Once again, a reminder to read all the information on your medication fact sheet, including side effects. It doesn't matter that it's been great for your friend, brother, Mum or aunty, it might NOT be right for you!

Chapter 2
Supplements

If we believed all the clever marketing spiel from the manufacturers, we would keel over and die if we didn't invest in a host of wonderful vitamins and antioxidants all delivered in neat packaging with fancy labels, usually with names and images designed to target and influence our subconscious mind. Good job they haven't met my Dad then – 94 years old, still playing golf three times a week and never had a supplement in his life. Looking at facts, your body requires at least 40 different minerals and they each play a major role in the immune response. Although our recommended dietary intake (RDI) varies with our different ages and stages of life, we should still ideally get all the vitamins and minerals we need from the food we eat. However poor soil quality, food intolerances and digestive issues often prevent this happening, and that's where supplements can play a crucial role.

That said, you can have too much of a good thing. Over supplementing is extremely common. I could cry when I see the amount of money that some people are investing in very good products will do nothing for them because they don't need them! Most times, the supplement will simply pass through the body and not do any harm if it isn't needed. The only damage that has been done is to the bank balance of the unfortunate soul who is only trying to be as healthy as they can but got sucked in by clever marketing. More worrying, is when people are taking supplements that are harming them.

Case Study

Jill, a healthy, active 66-year-old was developing macular degeneration (an age-related eye condition resulting in blurred or no vision). Jill was under the care of an ophthalmologist who had prescribed two supplements to support her eye health. He warned that her condition was serious and that she was in danger of losing her driving licence if the deterioration continued at the pace it was. Jill was understandably shaken and set about to help herself as much as she could by researching the condition.

Her best friend helpfully told her about a relative with a similar condition, who was taking an over-the-counter supplement he had found very beneficial, so Jill purchased some for herself. Concerned that she would lose her eyesight, Jill also went online and found a company in America who had produced an amazing product for eyes – the testimonials were glowing. Featuring people just like her, walking on sunny beaches and playing in parks with their grandchildren, the product promised perfect sight in older age. Well, of course Jill had to have several tubs of this marvellous creation. When Jill's daughter came to visit, she brought her another supplement that had proven antioxidants to work for macular degeneration, so Jill added that to her ever-increasing collection.

As the weeks went by, Jill was feeling increasingly unwell. Concerned by her condition, her daughter (an existing client of mine) suggested she came to see me. Despite living 5 hours away (and not wishing to Skype) Jill agreed to come along for a consultation. I had recommended that she brought along her recent blood test results so that I could see if they held any clues – and boy, did they! Her liver function was all over the place – clearly not at all happy. Jill said that her doctor had asked if she was drinking as he was also concerned by her liver results. She reported that she wasn't drinking at all as she was feeling so unwell. When I went through her supplements, the answer was staring me in the face ... vitamin A overload!

The upper limit of the recommended daily allowance (RDA) is 3,000 mcg. Jill was taking over 20,000 mcg! The liver is the main organ responsible for the storage, metabolism and distribution of vitamin A to peripheral tissues. Taking high doses of vitamin A can cause liver damage. No wonder her poor liver was waving a surrender flag! By the time I had finished Jill's consultation, she was left with one supplement (one of the originals her ophthalmologist had given her) and I recommended that she spread tomato puree on crackers every day with some hummus, and have that for lunch. Cooked tomatoes contain lycopene and lutein, crucial antioxidants to nourish and protect eye health.

I first saw Jill in July and by November she called to say that she was feeling 100% and that her recent eye test showed 20/20 vision in one eye and the other improving drastically. She was thrilled to bits! No danger of her losing her driving licence let alone her eyesight.

Then there was lovely Alison who had been prescribed vitamin D as her blood test had highlighted she was low in this important vitamin. So Alison took her vitamin D religiously year after year ... after year, after year ... and neither she nor the person who originally prescribed it (who had since retired) ever checked her levels. Too much vitamin D can cause problems such as constipation, nausea, headaches, fatigue and, in more serious cases, kidney stones and kidney damage. There is also a rare and serious condition called hypervitaminosis D which is directly caused by large doses of vitamin D from supplements (not by diet or sun exposure).

Whilst on the subject of vitamin D, I was visiting my new-born granddaughter Jessica, when the health visitor arrived. She asked Jenny, Jessica's mum, if she had taken advantage of the free vitamin drops being given away at the clinic. "She can have them until she's 5 years old", the health visitor happily announced. That's very good, providing the baby/child needs it. I asked what monitoring was done. The health visitor smiled and enthusiastically announced that "they can have as much as they want!" That wasn't actually my point.

It worries me to think that mothers who are being given free vitamins for their baby/toddler/young children might perhaps think that adding it copiously to the child's diet is beneficial. However, they could actually overdose their child. Symptoms of vitamin D overload are quite obscure (as earlier described), and I wonder how many babies and young children are being taken to the doctor with these 'ongoing ailments" and no link will be made with the vitamin D consumption. The child will no doubt be given superfluous medications to address the symptoms ... sigh.

If you are investing in supplements, please be careful. If you are buying online or having them delivered to you on a rolling contract, ask yourself, does the seller know if you are already taking other supplements? Do they know if you are taking any medications? Are they aware that you might have an underlying health condition that you are now masking with the supplement? I worry that people are unwittingly harming themselves and no-one will ever be held accountable.

Here are symptoms to watch out for:

Supplement	Overload symptoms
Vitamin A	Liver problems, birth defects
Vitamin D	Headaches, fatigue, constipation, nausea, kidney damage
Vitamin E	Decreased bone mass
Vitamin C	Diarrhoea, vomiting, nausea, headache, stomach cramps, heartburn, insomnia
Iron	Constipation, nausea, stomach ache, liver and heart issues

I am not a fan of multivitamins. If you are indeed deficient in specific nutrients, then focus on those and get the levels you need. Then, when your nutritional bank has been replenished, you should start weaning off. Certainly, in my clinics I make sure that my clients are getting what they need, when they need it (indeed IF they need it!), and then we monitor the impact, ensure the diet contains foods rich in the nutrients they need, and then we eventually wean off, assessing the body's response all the time. If we consider supplements performing for your body in the same way as stabilisers on a bike, if you take them away too soon, the body may wobble and weaken, but if you gradually cut back, either missing a day or lowering the dose, then your transition should be seamless.

Here are some of the most commonly used supplements and what they can do for you.

Probiotics

These strengthen your microflora, which in turn will help the absorption of nutrients from the food you eat (see pages 27–29 for specific species)

Magnesium

Magnesium is a mineral used in building bones, manufacturing proteins, releasing energy from muscle storage and regulating body temperature. Deficiencies of this mineral have been related to fluid retention, heart abnormalities and even to heart attacks. It is known for:

- **Boosting your spirits – magnesium deficiency causes a shortage of dopamine, the chemical found in the brain that regulates mood.**
- **Regulating your body temperature**
- **Relieving the cramps in your muscles**
- **Soothing your sinuses (and related headaches)**
- **Preventing inflammation in your mucous lining**

- Helping you cope with periods of stress
- Easing symptoms of endometriosis
- Easing any pre-menstrual symptoms you may experience, both physical and emotional
- Easing any tightness in your muscles
- Helping prevent migraines
- Transporting calcium to your bones
- Aiding weight loss by preventing cravings for sweet foods.

NB: If you are taking diuretics, they will decrease the magnesium stores in your body

Evening Primrose Oil

Perhaps best known and most widely used to ease pre-menstrual tension and assist hormonal imbalances, evening primrose oil can also clear skin, strengthen hair and nails and boost immune function. It can also help ease symptoms of arthritis.

Zinc

Zinc is a vital mineral for cholesterol balance, insulin production, immunity, smell and taste. A significant amount of zinc is lost through perspiration. Signs of deficiency include mood swings (including depression), loss of sex drive, fungal infections and ridges on the nails. Taking this mineral will:

- Prevent itchiness of the scalp
- Protect hair follicles and stimulate new growth
- Prevent thrush
- Prevent mouth ulcers, cold sores and bleeding gums
- Provide a boost for your immune system
- Help fight harmful yeasts in your system
- Help clear/prevent skin conditions such as acne by boosting cell renewal

- Help improve concentration and memory
- Help you process carbohydrates, fats and protein more efficiently
- Support prostate health.

Studies have shown that many people with Parkinson's disease are deficient in this mineral.

Omega-3

There are 2 sub-types of omega-3: DHA (docosahexaenoic acid) and EPA (eicosapentaenoic acid). DHA promotes cognitive function and this help with concentration and memory, whilst EPA helps alleviate pain and inflammation. Once you know why you are taking it, check the label to make sure you are getting the right dose. I once saw a client who was taking a product giving her 90 mg of EPA. She left my clinic with one providing 2000 mg.

Omega-3 can:

- Help reduce joint pain and improve motility
- Boost your immune system
- Help prevent dry skin
- Strengthen your bone tissue
- Eliminate toxins from your system
- Reduce inflammation throughout your body
- Stimulate the secretion of the appetite suppressant hormone leptin, which will help with weight loss
- Help prevent skin cancer
- Shrink precancerous polyps in the bowel.

Co-enzyme Q10

One of my personal favourites, CoQ10 is an antioxidant that your body produces naturally. Your cells use it for growth and maintenance, but levels decrease as you age.

Co-enzyme Q10 can:

- Boost metabolism
- Aid weight loss
- Help reduce hay fever symptoms
- Help with Parkinson's disease
- Increase sperm count
- Help prevent migraines
- Support the spleen and lymphatic system (boosting immunity)
- Increase your skin cells' capacity to produce vitamin D and is therefore helpful in the prevention of skin cancer.

(Before I studied nutrition, I had a basal cell carcinoma [bcc] appearing on my upper lip. It had been there a while and I was covering it with make-up, waiting for an appointment to have it removed. It vanished within a week of me taking a strong CoQ10 supplement.)

Vitamin B Complex

This popular group offers many benefits.

- B1 (thiamine) will help your nerves, digestive system and heart.
- B2 (riboflavin) will help prevent migraines and boost your energy.
- B3 (niacin) will support all your digestive organs, boost your circulation and prevent dizzy spells.
- B5 (pantothenic acid) will support your adrenal glands; help prevent hair loss; help prevent acne; help your system cope with allergies; support your respiratory system; help with ADHD, autism and depression; and fight harmful yeasts and urinary tract infections. Other conditions that could benefit from the use of B5 include dandruff, heart disease, carpal tunnel syndrome, respiratory problems, coeliac disease and diabetes.

- **B6 (pyridoxine) will support your kidneys and help balance your hormones. It also converts tryptophan to serotonin (tryptophan is an essential amino acid used for our nervous system, sleeping patterns, relaxation and mood), thus helping with depression.**
- **B12 (cyanocobalamin) will support your stomach acids and help boost your energy. Can also help prevent burning tongue and pins and needles and/or numbness in the extremities (but see overload and interactions below).**

Chromium

Chromium can help balance your blood sugars and support your pancreas. It can help satisfy sweet cravings, assist weight loss and protect you from type 2 diabetes. It is found naturally in foods such as eggs, whole grains, chicken, green capsicum and spinach.

Curcumin (a Derivate of Turmeric)

Curcumin can help reduce pain and inflammation in your bones and muscles.

Supplements and Interaction

Supplement	Interactions/overload symptoms
Vitamin E	Can interfere with absorption of medications, such as the antidepressants imipramine, nortriptyline and desimpramine; beta-blockers for high blood pressure, such as propranolol; antipsychotic medications, such as chlorpromazine; and cholesterol-lowering medications such as cholestyramine, colestipol, lovastatin, atorvastatin and pravastatin. Other types of interactions may occur, such as reducing the effectiveness of cyclosporine used for cancer treatment and mebendazole used for intestinal worm treatment. Always check with your health practitioner or pharmacist before you take vitamin E supplements.
Vitamin B12	There are conflicts between this vitamin and medications to reduce stomach acid, such as cimetidine, ranitidine, famotidine, omeprazole, esomeprazole and lansprazole; anticonvulsants, such as phenobarbital and phenytoin; chemotherapy agents, such as methotrexate; and cholesterol-lowering medications, such as cholestyramine, colsevelam and colestipol. Some antibiotics, such as tetracycline, should not be taken at the same time as vitamin B12.
Vitamin A	Having too much vitamin A from supplements or medications can cause dizziness, nausea, headaches, coma and even death. It can also cause birth defects. Many pregnant women take extra vitamins believing they are doing the best for their baby but it's very common for them to overload, especially in this vitamin.
Vitamin D	An interesting one because vitamin D overload symptoms are quite similar to deficiency symptoms; fatigue, nausea, headaches and bone pain are amongst them
Selenium	Not be taken if you have heart, liver or kidney disease.

Chapter 3
Eating Well

Children's Nutrition

The Basics

Before mealtimes, make sure the environment (physical and emotional) is as stable and calm as can be. Eating should be an enjoyable experience.

Watch that smaller children are chewing their food properly – there are no sharp teeth or cutting tools inside the digestive tract. Large chunks of undigested food can get 'stuck' in the intestines and cause pain, gas and bloating

Be mindful if your child continually repels a particular food – they might be intolerant to it. Inherently we know what is good or bad for us and children are more in tune with this inbuilt knowledge. Don't force them to eat anything they are averse to. A food and symptom diary can help identify food intolerances and allergies.

Probiotics and fermented foods will boost absorption of nutrients and aid digestion.

Breastfeeding

If your baby is having nothing other than breast milk but has digestive disturbances or seems unsettled all the time, consider checking for your OWN intolerances. Antibodies will travel through breastmilk. Also check for tongue-tie.

Babies

There is no hard and fast rule about when to wean your baby, although the average age is around 4 months. Foods eaten at this age are feeding the cells and influencing metabolic programming, immunity and long-term weight. Rice cereal mixed with breast milk (or formula), banana, pureed vegetables and cooked buckwheat groats are good introductory foods. Avoid honey and nuts as tiny digestive systems are not robust enough to digest these easily.

Infants and Toddlers

Good fats are very important at this development stage: avocado, coconut, oily fish. Omega-3 from fish is crucial for brain, behaviour, mood and skin and eye health. Use a good supplement if oily fish isn't liked – look for high EPA and DHA content (you'll find this on the label).

5–11-Year-Olds

Growth and energy is the focus here, so a good mix of proteins and carbohydrates is required for both. Roast dinners, spaghetti bolognese, fish and rice are good examples. Homemade is always best of course – try to resist packets and jars.

12–early Teens

Hormones are changing at this age! Zinc for your boys is paramount now. Good sources are oily fish and pumpkin seeds, but a supplement would be beneficial (around 25 mg a day but increase if acne is an issue). Girls need iodine for hormonal balance, together with iron. Spirulina, kelp, seaweed, etc. are very beneficial.

Vegetarian Considerations

A vegetarian diet can be very healthy. However, there are obvious nutrients that are likely to be depleted when meat is excluded, mainly iron, zinc and vitamin B12. If milk is also being excluded, then calcium levels are also at risk of becoming depleted.

Zinc is an essential mineral for proper growth of children and especially important through puberty. Zinc is also found in whole grains, brown rice, legumes and spinach.

Many vegetables like broccoli, sweet potatoes, great northern and navy beans, and leafy greens contain calcium. For children, soy milk or orange juice that is fortified with extra calcium can help them grow strong and fit. Cereals, bread, rice, and pasta that are fortified with iron should be consumed as most of the vegetarian foods are not a high source of iron.

As a vegetarian, you need to be aware of the importance of choosing a combination of plant foods (i.e. legumes [pulses], grains, seeds and nuts) to ensure protein balance and boost your energy. This is because plant-based foods are incomplete proteins and do not contain sufficient essential amino acids. By combining them you will form a higher quality protein.

Examples of combined proteins:

- **Lentils and rice (pulse and grain)**
- **Walnut, lentil and silverbeet loaf (nut, pulse and green vegetable)**
- **Tofu and vegetable stir fry with nuts (pulse, grain and nuts)**
- **Quinoa-stuffed capsicums (pulse, veg and grain).**

Vitamin B12 is naturally found in animal protein so you need to ensure that you actively seek to get this important vitamin from other sources such as fortified[1] cereals and drinks.

Portion Sizes (Intolerances Excepted)

I don't like to get too hung up on portion sizes; food should be enjoyed, not weighed and measured. However, as we now know, you can have too much of a good thing. I saw a sales rep once who spent most of his working day driving from one appointment to another. He was stopping at cafes or fast-food

1. 'Fortified' foods are those that have had nutrients added.

drive-throughs and was paying the penalty of an overload of pies, pizzas and burgers. We discussed his lifestyle and ran through some healthier options, even if that meant still calling in for takeaways. He found he could enjoy them, but reduced his portion sizes, cholesterol and waistline!

To help you gauge portions, here are some examples of a single portion size:

- 1 apple/1 banana/1 orange or fruit of a similar size
- 2 plums or other fruit of a similar size
- ½ a grapefruit or avocado
- 3 heaped tablespoons of vegetables (organic, fresh or frozen)
- 3 heaped tablespoons of fruit salad (organic, fresh or frozen)
- ½ cup of dried fruit (such as raisins and apricots)
- 1 handful of grapes, cherries or berries
- 1 dessert bowl of salad
- 150 ml glass of fruit juice (juicing your own will avoid harmful sugars, additives and preservatives)
- 150 g carton of yoghurt
- 4 cm cube of cheddar cheese
- 2 tbsp of cottage cheese
- A palm-sized portion of lean meat or fish.

Food as Medicine

Now that you have a fully efficient digestive system, take a look at the wonderful foods that it can now digest and feed to your cells. All foods have medicinal and healing properties, so before you reach for the medicine cabinet, why not invest in some healing foods instead?

Always try to buy fresh, seasonal produce. When it's not in season, frozen, dried or tinned would be your next choice (in that order).

Fruits and Nuts	Nutritional Content Includes:	Health Benefits Include:
Apples	Magnesium, calcium, vitamin C, pectin, beta-carotene, fibre, quercetin, chromium	Lower cholesterol Replenish healthy bacteria and relieve constipation Help remove toxins from your system Reduce risk of breast cancer
Apricots	High in iron, vitamin C, beta-carotene, B vitamins, iodine, folic acid, fibre, quercetin, calcium	Improve circulation Encourage bowel movements Support adrenal glands Help prevent anaemia
Avocados	Omega-3 and 6, vitamin C, B vitamins, potassium, magnesium, beta-carotene, folic acid, high in vitamin E, iron, vitamin K	Strengthen muscles Keep joints flexible Heal external and internal scarring Help prevent oral cancer Lower cholesterol and regulate blood pressure Protect against breast cancer
Bananas	Potassium, vitamin C, beta-carotene, vitamin B6, chromium, selenium, iron	Remove toxic metals Help control fluid balance Calm nerves and aid sleep Natural antacid for heartburn Encourage healthy bacteria

Fruits and Nuts	Nutritional Content Includes:	Health Benefits Include:
Berries (incl. strawberries, blueberries, raspberries, blackberries)	Iron, vitamin C, beta-carotene, quercetin	Boost immune system Help circulation Relieve menstrual cramps Strawberries lower LDL and increase HDL cholesterol Inhibit tumour growth by killing cancer cells
Cherries	Magnesium, calcium, phosphorous, vitamin C, fibre, potassium, iron.	Help prevent headaches and migraines Fight gout and arthritis
Coconut	Protein, natural sugars, palmitic acid, iron	Prevent constipation Help stop sweet cravings Aid weight loss Support thyroid function Lower bad cholesterol
Cranberries	Vitamin C, beta-carotene, potassium, quercetin	Support the respiratory system Kill bacteria and viruses in the kidneys, bladder and urinary tract. Support prostate health
Cucumber (for swollen hands and feet, put the skin in hot water and sip when cool enough to drink)	Vitamin C, vitamin A, magnesium, potassium, fibre, beta-carotene, silica	Supports liver, stomach, spleen and pancreas Helps prevent kidney stones Prevents constipation Regulates blood pressure

Fruits and Nuts	Nutritional Content Includes:	Health Benefits Include:
		Soothes skin irritations and reduces swellings (due to the ascorbic acid and caffeic acid) Helps prevent conjunctivitis and blepharitis
Dates	Calcium, iron, vitamins A, D and B3, beta-carotene, selenium, magnesium, potassium	Support respiratory system Encourage bowel movements Help stop sugar cravings Support bone health Boost blood and circulation and prevent anaemia
Figs	Magnesium, phosphorous, calcium, beta-carotene, iron, vitamins A, B and C, potassium, copper, vitamin K	Help move sluggish bowels Great for bone health due to the very high calcium and copper content Help prevent outbreaks of psoriasis and eczema
Goji berries	Selenium, vitamin C, EFAs, B vitamins, beta-carotene, iron	Boost energy Improve libido Help fight cancer Assist weight loss Improve concentration and memory Improve eyesight

Fruits and Nuts	Nutritional Content Includes:	Health Benefits Include:
Grapes	Magnesium, vitamin A, vitamin C, iron, calcium, fibre, chromium, potassium, vitamin B6, quercetin	Help keep cancer at bay Stimulate immune system Prevent heart disease Support liver function Help bones and joints
Grapefruit (avoid if taking blood pressure medication)	Calcium, magnesium, potassium, vitamin C, quercetin	Boost immune system Assist weight loss (they have fat burning enzymes) Support cardiovascular health Help detoxification Prevent/soothe mouth and throat infections
Kiwi fruit	Magnesium, phosphorous, vitamin C, vitamin E, potassium	Digestive enzymes to support stomach Remove excess sodium Encourage bowel movements
Lemons and limes	High in iron, vitamin C, potassium, quercetin	Support liver and gall bladder Help dissolve gallstones Boost immune system
Mangoes	Vitamin C, beta-carotene, vitamin B1 and B6, vitamin A, potassium	Great for kidney health Aid digestion Detoxify blood

Fruits and Nuts	Nutritional Content Includes:	Health Benefits Include:
Melons (best choice as a starter for a meal if watching your weight)	Calcium, magnesium, potassium, beta-carotene, vitamin C, phosphorous, chromium	Easily digested Support kidneys and bowel Lower cholesterol Ease arthritic pain Help lower risk of prostate cancer
Oranges	Calcium, potassium, beta-carotene, chromium, folic acid, vitamin C	Boost immune system Lower cholesterol Support endocrine and reproductive systems Encourage bowel movements
Papayas	Fibre, calcium, iron, magnesium, phosphorous, potassium, zinc, vitamin C, B vitamins, folic acid, vitamin E, beta-carotene	Support digestive health Help prevent bloating and gas
Passion fruit	Vitamin A, vitamin C, potassium, iron, B vitamin complex	Support respiratory health
Peaches (and nectarines)	Calcium, magnesium, folic acid, potassium, vitamin C, vitamin B3, fibre	Support kidneys and bladder. Encourage bowel movements. Protect eye health

Fruits and Nuts	Nutritional Content Includes:	Health Benefits Include:
Pears	Folic acid, calcium, magnesium, beta-carotene, potassium, iodine, pectin, quercetin	Support kidney and bladder function Help prevent urinary tract infections Support kidneys and bladder Encourage bowel movements Boost energy Detoxify Support eye health Support prostate health
Persimmons	Iron, vitamin C	Support thyroid function Aid digestion Help prevent psoriasis Soften and remove gallstones
Pineapples	Manganese, calcium, phosphorous, beta-carotene, potassium	Support your spleen and lymphatic system Support pancreas Soothe inflammation in mucous lining
Plums	Calcium, magnesium, potassium, phosphorous, rutin, vitamin C, B vitamins, manganese, selenium, chromium	Support your stomach acids Help reduce inflammation Help prevent psoriasis
Pomegranates	Vitamin C, B vitamins, phosphorous, calcium	Boost immune system Improve eye health Encourage bowel movements

Fruits and Nuts	Nutritional Content Includes:	Health Benefits Include:
Prunes	Calcium, phosphorous, potassium, beta-carotene, folic acid, vitamin B12	Support kidney and bladder function Boost immune system Boost concentration and memory – great brain food!
Nuts (fresh and unsalted)	Calcium, iron, potassium, magnesium, zinc, selenium, omega-3, vitamin	Lower cholesterol Relieve constipation Prevent psoriasis Just two Brazil nuts will provide your daily selenium requirement Walnuts are rich in omega-3 and help ease arthritic pain Almonds aid digestion, help protect against osteoarthritis and lower cholesterol Cashew nuts are rich in protein and iron (but high in calories!) Hazelnuts have a lower fat content than most other nuts Pecans are high in calcium Peanuts help endometriosis

Fruits and Nuts	Nutritional Content Includes:	Health Benefits Include:
Tangerines (and tangelos and mandarins)	B vitamins, calcium, potassium, zinc, pectin	Aid digestion Support adrenal function Boost immune system
Tomatoes	Vitamin C, vitamin A, folic acid, calcium, magnesium, chromium, phosphorous, fibre, vitamin E	Reduce liver inflammation Support eye health Support prostate gland

Vegetables, Pulses and Legumes	Nutritional Content Includes:	Health Benefits Include:
Asparagus	Potassium, folic acid, beta-carotene, vitamin C	Supports kidneys and adrenal glands Encourages healthy bacteria
Aubergine/eggplant	Calcium, beta-carotene, folic acid	Prevents strokes and haemorrhages Protects arteries from cholesterol damage
Barley	B vitamins, magnesium, zinc	Lowers cholesterol Supports liver and spleen Aids sleep Helps prevent premenstrual syndrome
Beetroot	Potassium, magnesium, iron, vitamin C, folic acid, fibre, potassium, folic acid	Supports liver, gall bladder and spleen Good for skin conditions Helps prevent anaemia
Bok Choy	Vitamin A, vitamin C, B vitamins (high in B6), vitamin K, calcium, phosphorous, potassium, manganese, lutein, lycopene, iron, magnesium	Boosts immune system Encourages bowel movements Lowers cholesterol Supports eye health

Vegetables, Pulses and Legumes	Nutritional Content Includes:	Health Benefits Include:
Broccoli	Vitamins B2, B3 and B5, vitamin C, vitamin K, folic acid, beta-carotene, magnesium, chromium, calcium, co-enzyme Q10	Cleanses intestines and supports bowel movements Boosts metabolism and energy Supports eye health Eases endometriosis pain
Brussel sprouts	Calcium, magnesium, iron, potassium, beta-carotene, folic acid, vitamin C, vitamin E, vitamin K	Support pancreatic function Help fight colon cancer Encourage bowel movements
Cabbage	Vitamins A,C and E, magnesium, folic acid, fibre, calcium, vitamin K, quercetin	Detoxifies the digestive system Aids digestion of fats Helps prevent osteoarthritis
Capsicum	Vitamins B and C, beta-carotene, potassium, folic acid	Lowers blood pressure Boosts circulation and immune system
Carrots	Magnesium, calcium, beta-carotene, potassium, silica, iron	Support liver and kidneys Good for skin conditions Boost circulation Prevent anaemia
Cauliflower	Magnesium, calcium, beta-carotene, folic acid, vitamin K, potassium, quercetin	Support kidneys and bladder Lower blood pressure Help detoxify blood Support bowel Ease arthritis

Vegetables, Pulses and Legumes	Nutritional Content Includes:	Health Benefits Include:
Celeriac	Magnesium, potassium, calcium, vitamin C, vitamin K, phosphorous, manganese	Eases arthritis Supports kidney health Beneficial for nervous and lymphatic systems
Celery	Vitamin B3, beta-carotene, folic acid, potassium, quercetin	Aids digestion Supports adrenal glands Helps prevent migraines Eases arthritis Lowers blood pressure
Chickpeas	High in folic acid, iron, calcium	Aid digestion Boost energy
Corn	Iron, magnesium, potassium, vitamin B3, zinc	Great for heart health Prevents neural-tube birth defects Prevents constipation and haemorrhoids
Dark green leafy vegetables, particularly spinach	Iron, B vitamins, potassium, chromium, magnesium, vitamin E, quercetin, phyto-oestrogens, manganese	Increase iron supplies Balance hormones Support digestive health Encourage regular bowel movements
Fennel	Calcium, magnesium, folic acid, vitamin C, phyto-oestrogens, fibre	Aids digestion of fats Balances hormones Supports spleen and lymphatic system If breastfeeding, it will help your baby's digestive system and prevent colic

Vegetables, Pulses and Legumes	Nutritional Content Includes:	Health Benefits Include:
Flax seeds	Omega-3 essential fatty acids, vitamin E	Detoxifies blood Supports bones and muscles Balances hormones Prevent constipation
Garlic	Calcium, potassium, vitamin C, phosphorous, silica	Lowers cholesterol Kills harmful yeasts and encourages healthy gut bacteria Balances hormones Supports sinuses Prevents fungal infections Boosts immune system
Kidney beans	Protein, magnesium, calcium, potassium	Lowers cholesterol Encourages healthy gut bacteria
Kumara/sweet potato	Calcium, magnesium, potassium, vitamin C, vitamin E, vitamin A	Eliminates heavy metal toxins
Leeks	Vitamin B3, potassium, calcium, folic acid, quercetin	Support regular bowel movements Encourage healthy gut bacteria
Lentils	Calcium, zinc , potassium, iron, B vitamins, magnesium, folic acid	Encourage healthy bacteria Support regular bowel movements Protect against heart disease and type 2 diabetes

Vegetables, Pulses and Legumes	Nutritional Content Includes:	Health Benefits Include:
Mung beans/aduki beans	Magnesium, iron, potassium, zinc, B vitamins, folic acid, silica	Boost circulation Detoxifying Bean sprouts help relieve endometriosis pain
Mushrooms	Selenium, calcium, iron, B vitamins (high in vitamin B12), folic acid, zinc, magnesium	Support immune system Lower cholesterol Ease arthritic pain Shitake mushrooms can limit the harmful side effects of chemotherapy
Noodles (rice noodles)	Protein, phosphorous, iron, selenium, potassium, minimal calcium, zinc, copper and manganese	Easily digested Energy boosting
Olives	Iron, calcium, beta-carotene, vitamin E, copper	Aid digestion Support liver and gall bladder Ease dermatitis and eczema Keep blood vessels healthy Good for bones

Vegetables, Pulses and Legumes	Nutritional Content Includes:	Health Benefits Include:
Onions	Potassium, magnesium, chromium, vitamins B3 and B6, vitamin E, vitamin C, silica, quercetin, folate	Detoxifying and antibiotic Encourage healthy bacteria Reduce high blood pressure Red onions contain quercetin – a powerful bioflavonoid that will protect prostate health
Peas	B vitamins, zinc, iron, folic acid, magnesium, calcium, potassium, vitamin K	Support liver function Reduce stomach cancer risk Boost immunity
Potatoes	Vitamins B3 and B6, vitamin C, folic acid, iron, chromium and potassium	Lower blood pressure Support for liver health Boost energy
Pumpkins	Magnesium, potassium, vitamin C, beta-carotene, iron, vitamin B6, magnesium	Help balance your blood sugar levels Pumpkin seeds support prostate health Boost immune system Support healthy skin and heart

Vegetables, Pulses and Legumes	Nutritional Content Includes:	Health Benefits Include:
Radishes	Calcium, magnesium, potassium, beta-carotene, silicon, iron, vitamin B6	Lower high blood pressure Support heart health Aid production of digestive juices Support liver and gall bladder
Rhubarb	Vitamin C, calcium, magnesium, phosphorous, potassium, beta-carotene,	Encourages bowel movements Helps balance your hormones Lowers cholesterol
Rocket	Vitamins A, B, C , K and E, zinc, iron, iodine, phosphorous	Stimulates digestion Protects from cancer Boosts immunity
Spirulina	Potassium, iodine, iron, vitamin B3, phosphorous, beta-carotene	Immune boosting Anti-inflammatory Supports digestive health Helps hay fever
Sesame seeds	Zinc, vitamin E, calcium, silica, protein, vitamin B3, iron	Boost immune system Lower cholesterol Anti-inflammatory Support adrenal glands
Sunflower seeds	Protein, B vitamins, EFAs, potassium, iron, magnesium, zinc, calcium	Detoxifying Encourage bowel movements Support adrenal glands Balance hormones

Vegetables, Pulses and Legumes	Nutritional Content Includes:	Health Benefits Include:
Turnips	Vitamin C, iron, calcium, vitamin B6, magnesium, iron, potassium	Support digestive health Ease symptoms of asthma and bronchitis Lower blood pressure
Watercress	Vitamin C, vitamin A, some B vitamins, iodine, iron, calcium, potassium, zinc	Detoxifying Supports adrenal glands Boosts immunity Supports healthy skin Promotes healthy thyroid function

Meats and Fish	Nutritional Content Includes:	Health Benefits Include:
Beef, including steaks – lean cuts	B vitamins, iron, zinc, chromium, selenium, B vitamins, magnesium, potassium	Can prevent anaemia Boosts energy Helps maintain muscle mass
Chicken – skinless	Vitamin B3, vitamin B6, vitamin B12, magnesium, potassium, iron, zinc, selenium, chromium	Supports spleen and lymphatic system Encourages healthy thyroid function Boosts energy
Duck	B vitamins, iron, zinc, selenium, omega-3, omega-6, vitamin K, vitamin E	Boosts immune system Supports thyroid health Protects bones Supports heart health
Fish – particularly the oily varieties such as salmon, mackerel and sardines	Omega-3 fatty acids, B vitamins, selenium, iron, zinc, iodine	Support bone and heart health Aid digestion Lower cholesterol Support healthy thyroid function Can help improve mood
Lamb	Protein, B vitamins, iron, zinc,	Can prevent anaemia Provides eight essential amino acids
Liver	Co-enzyme Q10, iron, protein, chromium, zinc, vitamin A, folic acid, B vitamins	Assists metabolism Boosts energy Can prevent anaemia Supports adrenal glands

Meats and Fish	Nutritional Content Includes:	Health Benefits Include:
Oysters	Zinc, vitamin B12, vitamin C, chromium, iron	Supports cardiovascular health Boost immune system Helps cognitive function
Pork	B vitamins, iron, magnesium, zinc, phosphorus, potassium, chromium, vitamin K	Promotes cell growth Improves muscle mass Boosts energy
Turkey	Vitamin B12, B6 , B3 iron, zinc, selenium, chromium, protein	Supports thyroid and prostate Boosts energy Aids sleep
Venison	Co-enzyme Q10B 12, B2, B3, B6, phosphorous, protein, selenium, iron, zinc	Boosts energy Can prevent anaemia Helps relieve migraines

Dairy	Nutritional Content Includes:	Health Benefits Include:
Cheese	Protein, calcium, B vitamins, vitamin K	Supports bone health Boosts energy
Milk – dairy	Calcium, phosphorous, vitamin B2, vitamin B12, protein	Boosts immune system Lifts mood
Yoghurt (choose probiotic varieties)	Calcium, protein, vitamin B2, potassium and vitamin D	Supports digestive health

Other	Nutritional Content Includes:	Health Benefits Include:
Aloe Vera	Contains all eight essential amino acids and eleven of the 14 'secondary' amino acids as well as Vitamins A, B1, B2, B6, B12, C and E	Aids digestion Boosts immune system Reduces inflammation
Amaranth (gluten free herb/grain)	Calcium, magnesium, iron, phosphorus, protein	Supports digestive health Prevents bowel problems. Strengthens respiratory system Lowers cholesterol
Bread – whole grain	Iron, calcium, B vitamins, fibre, chromium	Boosts energy Supports heart health Aids digestion Lowers cholesterol
Buckwheat (a herb that is used as a grain)	Folic acid, magnesium, manganese, calcium, vitamin B3, potassium, phosphorous, iron, calcium, rutin, tryptophan, fibre	Supports pancreatic function Aids digestion Boosts energy Helps circulation Promotes restful sleep
Carob	Calcium, B vitamins, phosphorous, iron, vitamin A	Lowers cholesterol Can help prevent anaemia Combats cancer

Other	Nutritional Content Includes:	Health Benefits Include:
Chia seeds – sprinkle on cereals and salads or mix with water and lemon for a healthy chia fresco drink	Protein, fibre, omega-3, calcium, iron, zinc, phosphorous, manganese	Lower blood pressure Lower cholesterol Support bowel and pancreas Support bone health
Eggs	Protein, vitamins B12, A, D and E, iron, phosphorous, chromium, zinc	Support heart health Boost energy Support bone health
Honey	Natural sugars (fructose and glucose), enzymes and amino acids, healthy bacteria	Improves digestive health Boosts circulation Stimulates re-growth of cells
Kelp	Iodine, calcium, potassium, magnesium, vitamin A, vitamin C, vitamin E, vitamin D and B complex	Boosts metabolism Supports kidney health
Lecithin	Choline, protein	Lowers cholesterol Excellent for cardiovascular health Supports liver Improves memory and concentration
Millet	Magnesium, iron, protein, fibre, silica, phosphorous	Boosts energy Aids digestion Aids weight loss

Other	Nutritional Content Includes:	Health Benefits Include:
Oats	Fibre, protein, magnesium, potassium, zinc, B vitamins	Lowers cholesterol Helps Type 2 diabetes Boosts mood
Pasta (whole wheat)	Iron, folic acid, iron, B vitamins	Boosts metabolism Supports heart health
Quinoa (pronounced keenwah) is a derivative of the spinach family but is used as a grain	Calcium, iron, magnesium, B-complex vitamins, folate, protein, fibre, potassium, manganese, nine essential amino acids	Excellent for digestive health Fights cancer Boosts energy
Rice (brown)	Calcium, iron, magnesium, potassium, zinc, fibre, manganese	Supports digestion Lowers cholesterol
Rye	Calcium, iron, magnesium, phosphorous, potassium, zinc, fibre, selenium, minimal amounts of vitamin C and B vitamins	Supports liver function Helps diabetes
Slippery Elm (available in supplement or powder form in health food shops and pharmacies)	A wealth of easily absorbed nutrients	Supports digestive health Reduces inflammation

Other	Nutritional Content Includes:	Health Benefits Include:
Spelt	Protein	To support your digestive function, particularly your bowel
Tofu	Protein, iron, choline, fibre, tryptophan, manganese, magnesium, omega-3, selenium, phosphorous, calcium	To keep protein and iron intake up in the absence of a regular meat source
Wheatgrass	Chlorophyll, amino acids, enzymes, vitamins and minerals (high in magnesium)	To support your liver and bowel, encourage healthy bacteria and boost your immune system

Top Herbs and Spices

Alfalfa	This has unique properties that will help endometriosis.
Astragalus	To support your adrenal glands and help you cope with stress.
Bilberry	To protect you from macular degeneration and cataracts.
Black Cohosh	This will balance your hormones, boost your circulation and lower cholesterol. Excellent for all menopausal symptoms (avoid if you have high blood pressure) – reduces facial and body hair, hot flushes, fatigue and mood swings.
Black pepper	To aid weight loss.
Bladderwrack (a form of kelp)	This will support your thyroid and adrenal glands and help with weight loss.
Cayenne	To support your spleen and your lymphatic system. It will also help stop haemorrhoids by stabilising the circulation to the anus. Can also help prevent varicose veins.
Cinnamon	This has unique anti-inflammatory properties that will help relive/prevent rheumatism. It will help your body's response to insulin and prevent type-2 diabetes. Aids weight loss.
Coriander	Its leaves contain antihistamines that help reduce allergy symptoms.
Cumin	This will aid your digestion and prevent gas and indigestion. It can help carpal tunnel syndrome.
Feverfew	This will help prevent migraines as it prevents constriction of blood vessels in the brain

Ginger	To improve your circulation, boost your immune system and support your digestive juices. Eases arthritis, rheumatism and muscle spasms. Loosens phlegm and therefore helps asthma, bronchitis and respiratory problems.
Gingko	This can prevent some of the symptoms of health deterioration associated with aging, such as Alzheimer's, memory loss, loss of hearing and eyesight deterioration. Ginkgo also helps prevent blood clotting.
Ginseng	To help your liver break own fats more efficiently and aid weight loss.
Gotu Kola	One of the most important rejuvenative herbs in Ayurvedic medicine. The main revitalising herb for nerves and brain cells.
Marjoram (and oregano)	To help relieve ear, nose, throat and lung infections.
Marshmallow Root	To manage the acid/alkaline balance of your bowel and flush out excess mucous.
Milk thistle	To support hormones, liver, adrenal glands and bowel.
Mint	To support your digestive organs and aid weight loss
Parsley	This is particularly effective at easing indigestion and menstruation problems. It will also balance the fluid levels in your body.
Peppermint	To aid digestion and support your sinuses.
Turmeric	To lower your blood pressure and cholesterol, boost your immune system and protect you from heart disease. It has amazing anti-inflammatory properties and will keep all your cells healthy. Known to help dissolve gallstones.

And Finally...

Armed with all this precious knowledge, here are some ideas for further investing in your health.

TAKE CONTROL

It's your life and every day matters. Consider the following:

- Blood tests – request a test to cover basics such as cholesterol, blood glucose, complete blood count and liver function. If your energy is low, ask for a full iron profile, B12, full blood count and thyroid function. If you've been unwell for some time, yet blood tests have revealed nothing out of the ordinary, it's worth asking for an ANA (anti-nuclear antibodies) test to check for autoimmune conditions. If your doctor is reluctant to help in this regard, there are private testing centres. Keep copies of your results in order to track and monitor your progress. Many doctors' surgeries have online patient portals where you can access all your records.
- Food intolerance test – there are many ways to test for intolerances. Go with the method you are most comfortable with.
- A personal health and nutrition assessment – generic 'diets' cannot take account of your unique personal needs. Your past and current health, stress, sleep, hormonal changes, digestive health, hereditary conditions, food intolerances and more should be thoroughly investigated to ensure you are eating foods that are nourishing and supporting you.
- Check the side effects of medications – please, please do!
- Keep a food and symptom diary (see Appendix 9, 210–211). Recording what and when you eat and drink, alongside how you are feeling, your energy, skin, digestion, sleep, etc., can be very insightful.

Appendix 1
Tips for Weight Loss

Whilst your focus should always be on your health, there are some practical things you can do to aid weight loss if that is one of your goals.

Weight gain happens for a variety of reasons including genetics (yes, really!), lifestyle, stress, lack of exercise, food intolerances, nutritional deficiencies, a weak digestive system, overeating, poor food choices, hormonal imbalances, medication side-effects and many more reasons besides. Don't look for quick fixes and sudden drastic weight-loss results. If you lose weight too quickly, it will only be temporary, and you are likely to gain it all back – and more – due to the imbalances you have forced on your body.

Here are simple, manageable things you can do to boost your metabolism and your energy, which will lead to sustainable and permanent weight loss.

- Start your day with a cup of hot water and lemon. This will cleanse your digestive tract, boost your immune system and help to energise you.
- Have a probiotic. Research has proven that increasing the healthy bacteria in your intestines leads to better absorption of nutrients throughout the day – and that leads to weight loss! The species *Lactobacillus lantis* has been identified as particularly useful for weight loss and is missing in many overweight people.
- Take apple cider vinegar. Taking 2 teaspoons of apple cider vinegar in a small glass of water, 20 minutes before your meal, will aid digestion, balance blood glucose levels and aid weight loss.

- Add seeds to breakfasts and salads – they are low calorie and highly nutritious and help boost your energy.
- Snack on fruit, nuts, and seeds. People who snack on fresh, unsalted nuts tend to lose weight more easily than those who do not. That's because nuts are high in protein and essential fatty acids and help keep you feeling full. One portion is 6–8 almonds, 2–3 Brazil nuts or 4–5 walnuts.
- Recognise hunger versus thirst; very often, thirst can feel like hunger. Sipping water regularly throughout the day carries nutrients to your cells and will help keep hunger pains at bay.
- Reduce carbohydrate intake in the evening. Carbohydrates (potatoes, pasta, rice, etc.) break down as sugars in the body for you to use as energy. If you don't burn the energy off, the sugars will be stored as fat.
- Don't skip meals. People who eat breakfast followed by small regular meals thereafter are generally slimmer than those who do not. Going without food for longer than 3 hours may get you to a point that when you do eat, your hunger causes you to eat the wrong food or too much of it!
- Eat slowly! Thoroughly chewing your food is not only beneficial for your digestive health, it is also a great weight loss tool. It takes about 20 minutes for your brain to register that you have had enough.
- Consider the Glycaemic Index. The Glycaemic Index measures the speed at which carbohydrates break down into sugar in our bodies. Low GI foods are digested slowly, keep you feeling fuller for longer and keep your blood glucose levels even. Sticking to mostly low to moderate GI foods will help weight loss (see pages 72–73).
- Avoid fried foods. Apart from stripping valuable nutrients, frying foods adds fat and calories. Stir-fry, bake and steam instead.
- Avoid unhealthy takeaways. These are usually high in fat and calories and the portion sizes are usually excessive. If you are out with friends and they have opted for fast food, choose salads, low fat Subway, crumbed fish (as opposed to fried), etc. Most fast-food outlets offer low fat alternatives.

- Watch your drink. Fizzy drinks, some fruit juices and alcoholic drinks are high in calories. For example, a 12-ounce can of Coca Cola contains 154 calories, an 8-ounce glass of lemonade can contain up to 110 calories, a 7-ounce gin and tonic is 171 calories and a 3-ounce glass of white wine is 70 calories. Don't be fooled by the 'diet' drinks either. Artificial sweeteners actually stimulate appetite, so although you may be getting fewer calories in your drink, you're likely to feel hungrier later. Instead, a glass of vegetable juice a day is highly nutritious and a great weight loss tool, or try two teaspoons of chia seeds in water with a little lemon. Lastly, avoid fizzy drinks, especially the 'energy' varieties!
- Avoid TV dinners. Research has proven that eating in front of the television results in a greater intake.
- Keep a food and exercise diary. It's useful to keep a food diary when you are trying to lose weight. You'll be able to see at a glance just how much you are sneaking in that you might not otherwise have been aware of, and identify where and when your weak spots may be. Even just having the odd bite of someone else's chocolate bar and accepting a chip or two can soon mount up.
- Use a list when shopping for food. Planning ahead is a great weight loss tool. Only buy what's on your list and do not shop (or write the list!) when you are hungry.
- Sleep in the dark. A study just published in the Proceedings of the National Academy of Sciences shows that you can gain weight just by sleeping with a dim light on (like the glow from a nightlight).
- Balance your hormones. Hormonal imbalances are often responsible for weight gain.
- Tune in to your circadian rhythm. Eating within a ten-hour time frame has been proven to aid weight management. Allow your body to settle before winding down for bed and to prevent stimulating your digestive system late at night, when it will store any unprocessed food as fat (midnight snackers beware!)

- **Check the side effects of medication. Many common medications list weight gain as a potential side effect, especially those prescribed for mood disorders. Take the time to read all side effects of any medications you are taking.**
- **Recognise success. NOT putting weight on is a success – losing it is a bonus!**

Appendix 2
Understanding Thyroid Results

Whether high or low, an abnormal Thyroid Stimulating Hormone (TSH) level indicates an excess or deficiency in the amount of thyroid hormone available to the body, but it does not indicate

TSH Range 0.4–4.0	Free T4 Range 9–25	Free or Total T3 Range 3.5–7.8	Probable Interpretation
High	Normal	Normal	Mild (subclinical) hypothyroidism
High	Low	Low or normal	Hypothyroidism
Low	Normal	Normal	Mild (subclinical) hyperthyroidism
Low	High or normal	High or normal	Hyperthyroidism
Low	Low or normal	Low or normal	Non-thyroidal illness, pituitary (secondary) hypothyroidism
Normal	High	High	Thyroid hormone resistance syndrome (a mutation in the thyroid hormone receptor decreases thyroid hormone function)

Hypothyroidism: Underactive thyroid.

Hyperthyroidism: Overactive thyroid.

the reason why. An abnormal TSH test result is usually followed by additional testing to investigate the cause of the increase or decrease. The table[1] opposite summarises some examples of typical test results and their potential meaning, but other factors affecting each individual should be taken into account.

1. From labtestsonline.

Appendix 3
Tyramine

Tyramine is an amino acid that occurs in many foods. Whilst the body should metabolise tyramine, some systems struggle and this can lead to health conditions, including migraines, a burning mouth and tongue, high blood pressure and panic attacks.

Tyramine amounts can vary among foods due to different processing, storage and preparation methods, but the following foods contain tyramine:

Fruit	Vegetables	Meat	Fish
Avocados	Aubergines/ Eggplant	Bacon	Caviar
Bananas	Broad beans	Corned beef	Herring
Coconuts		Ham	Smoked fish
Figs		Pepperoni	
Olives		Pork	
Pineapples		Salami	
Plums (red)		Sausage	
Raspberries		Pepperoni	

Misc	Dairy	Drinks
Caffeine	Blue cheese	Beer
Chocolate	Camembert	Liqueurs
Marmite/vegemite 'yeast' products	Cheddar	Sherry
Peanuts	Feta	Wine
Sauerkraut	Gorgonzola	
Soy sauce	Gouda	
Tempeh	Mozzarella	
Teriyaki sauce	Sour cream	
Tofu	Stilton	
	Swiss cheese	
	Mozzarella	
	Yoghurt	

If you're taking an MAOI antidepressant you should avoid/limit your intake of tyramine to avoid unwanted and potentially harmful side effects. Examples of MAOIs include isocarboxazid (Marplan), phenelzine (Nardil), selegiline (Emsam, Eldepryl, Zelapar) and tranylcypromine (Parnate).

Appendix 4

Meal Ideas to Fight Depression, Anxiety and Insomnia

Begin with a cup of hot water with lemon juice.

Take a probiotic (containing the strains *Lactobacillus helveticus* and *Lactobacillus rhamnosus*).

Breakfast: porridge oats.

Snacks: dates, nuts, bananas, cherries.

Lunch: Protein (e.g. tuna, eggs, tofu, salmon) with complex carbohydrates (e.g. pasta, brown rice).

Evening meal: chicken or turkey with vegetables.

Drink: water throughout the day and include herbal teas such as chamomile.

Suggested add-ins: probiotic yoghurt, fermented food (e.g. sauerkraut, kombucha, kimchee).

Every 'body' is different. The above suggestions offer a range of foods that contain the nutrients that can calm the mind and body.

If you introduce a new food, notice the effect it has on you, including digestion (e.g. burping, tummy ache, nausea). It is helpful to keep a food and symptom diary to track any changes (see Appendix 9, pages 220–221).

If taking supplements, be sure to read the label(s) so that you are taking them at the right time of day and with/without food as directed. Also check there's no clash with medications.

Appendix 5
Salicylates

Salicylates are natural chemical compounds made by all fruits and vegetables. Salicylates protect them against disease, fungal growth and insect attacks. There are a number of health benefits for us, and we've been using salicylate extracts medicinally for thousands of years. Aspirin is a good example of this. However, many people are sensitive to salicylates and it can cause a number of health issues including welts, headaches and ADHD. *NB: Do not follow a strictly low salicylate diet without advice from your health professional or you could be at risk of unnecessarily excluding vital nutrients.*

Fruit

Negligible	Low	Moderate	High	Very High
Bananas	Apples (Golden Delicious)	Apples (Red Delicious)	Apples (other varieties)	All dried fruits
Limes	Papaya	Custard apple	Cantaloupe	Apricots
Pears (ripe and peeled)		Figs (Canned or dried)	Cherries (canned Morello)	Avocados
		Lemons	Grapefruit	Blackberries
		Loquat	Kiwi fruit	Blackcurrants
		Mangoes	Lychee	Blueberries
				Boysenberries

Negligible	Low	Moderate	High	Very High
		Passion fruit	Mandarins	Cherries (all other kinds)
		Pears (canned)*	Melons (all other kinds)	Cranberries
		Pears (with peel)	Mulberry	Currants
		Persimmons	Nectarines	Dates
		Pomegranates	Peaches	Grapes
		Rhubarb	Sugar bananas	Guava
			Watermelon	Loganberries
				Oranges
				Melon (rock)
				Pineapple
				Plums
				Prunes
				Redcurrants
				Strawberries
				Sultanas
				Tangelos

*Canned pears have negligible amounts of salicylate if they are in sugar syrup, but if they are in natural juices/syrups, they have a moderate amount of salicylate as these often contain some peel, which contains salicylates.

Vegetables

Negligible	Low	Moderate	High	Very High
Bamboo shoots	Asparagus (fresh)	Asparagus (tinned)	Alfalfa sprouts	Capsicums/ sweet peppers
Beans (dried – not borlotti)	Beans (green)	Aubergine/ Eggplant	Artichokes	Champignon mushrooms
Cabbage (green or white)	Bean sprouts	Beetroot	Aubergine/ eggplant (with peel)	Chicory
Celery	Borlotti beans	Carrots	Broad beans	Chilli/hot peppers
Green split peas	Brussel sprouts	Lettuce (other than Iceberg)	Broccoli	Courgette/ zucchini
Lentils (brown)	Cabbage (red)	Marrows	Cucumbers	Endive
Lentils (red)	Cauliflower	Mushrooms	Okra	Gherkins
Lettuce (Iceberg)	Chickpeas	Olives (fresh black)	Olives (canned black)	Olives (canned green)
Peas (dried)	Chives	Parsnips	Radishes	Tomatoes
Potatoes (old/ white and peeled)	Leeks	Potatoes (new and red)	Spinach (fresh)	Tomato products
Swede	Mung bean sprouts	Pumpkin	Sweet potatoes/ kumara	Water Chestnut
	Onions	Snow peas	Watercress	
	Peas (green)	Spinach (frozen)		
	Potatoes (white with peel)			

Negligible	Low	Moderate	High	Very High
	Shallots	Sprouts		
	Yellow split peas	Sweetcorn		
		Turnip		

Nuts and Seeds

Negligible	Low	Moderate	High	Very High
Poppy seeds	Cashews	Desiccated coconut	Brazil nuts	Almonds
	Hazelnuts	Peanut butter	Macadamia nuts	Peanuts with skins on
	Pecans	Pumpkin seeds	Pine nuts	
	Sunflower seeds	Sesame seeds	Pistachios	
		Walnuts		

Appendix 6
Hints and Tips for Shift Workers

Identify the shift that you will be working well in advance so that you can plan your meals and snacks.

Eat according to the time of day rather than the time of your shift because the digestive system naturally slows down during the night. This makes food harder to digest, especially fats and sugars. If you are on an evening shift, have your main meal before you start.

Take your own food rather than rely on cafe or canteen choices. Cold meats and fish are good protein choices, bagels and wraps will digest more easily at night than sandwiches, and light carbohydrate foods such as cold rice or pasta salads will help sustain your energy.

Keep snacks nutritious rather than opting for chocolate, crisps, biscuits and cakes. Healthier options would be a handful of nuts, fruit, crackers, celery with peanut butter, dried fruit – and even a boiled egg!

Watch your drinks. Caffeine is a stimulant and stays in your system for 8 hours. If you drink it on your shift, you will have difficulty falling asleep after your shift finishes. Likewise, drinks such as V and Red Bull will interrupt your sleep patterns. Better choices are water (of course!), fruit juice, smoothies, decaffeinated tea and coffee, herbal teas and green tea.

Try and exercise during your shift – even gentle stretching exercises. This not only keeps you alert, it helps massage the digestive organs, prevents indigestion and will help regulate your sleep patterns.

Chew your food thoroughly before you swallow. (A common problem for shift workers is that they become too hungry and tend to eat far too quickly!) You have no sharp teeth or cutting tools inside your digestive tract. If your teeth don't do a good job, your digestive organs will struggle and foods that can't be processed by your gastric juices will be stored as fat and/or toxic waste. Chewing also stimulates production of stomach acid. The only part of digestion you have control over is chewing – so do a good job!

Eat little and often to sustain your energy, regulate your blood sugar levels and promote a healthy digestive system. Don't go any longer than 3 hours without eating.

Remember you are unique and whilst the above is general advice for anyone working shifts, your body will have specific needs (male, female, health conditions, stage of life etc.).

Appendix 7
Oestrogen Level Score Chart[1]

Oestrogen is a fluctuating hormone. Low levels are common in women approaching menopause.

Symptom	Score
Mood changes/depression	
Anxiety or irritability	
Poor concentration and memory	
Poor sleeping patterns	
Fatigue	
Headaches	
Hot flushes	
Lightheadedness	
Joint pain	
Increase in facial hair	
Dry skin – sudden increase in wrinkles	
Crawling sensation in the skin	
Burning feet	
Loss of libido	
Vaginal dryness	
TOTAL	

The symptoms opposite are characteristic of Oestrogen deficiency. Rate the severity of each symptom as you experience it, then total the combined scores.

Absent = 0 Mild = 1 Moderate = 2 Severe = 3

Results

0–10	10–15	16–30	Over 30
Oestrogen levels appear to be stable	Oestrogen levels could be declining	Likely oestrogen deficient	You need oestrogen!

Over 30: You appear to be VERY deficient in oestrogen. A blood test is recommended to check your levels of oestradiol (the strongest oestrogen hormone), progesterone and also follicle-stimulating hormone (FSH).

1. This chart is adapted from a questionnaire devised by Professor Chris Nordin, Institute of Medical and Veterinary Science, Adelaide University, South Australia.

Appendix 8
Pregnancy Trimesters

Pregnancy is a special time, and each and woman will experience it in her own way. It brings many changes in the body, so 'feeding your cells' has never been more important! This appendix offers generic advice, but everyone is different. It is therefore beneficial to have a personal health and nutrition assessment to get specific advice for your individual needs.

The following nutrients are particularly important for the growth and development of your baby and to keep your body healthy and energised. You can also focus on specific needs for each trimester. Underpinning these, it's helpful to invest in a probiotic to boost immunity, aid absorption of nutrients and reduce nausea and sickness. There are products designed specifically for pregnancy.

1st Trimester: This is the most critical stage of development when the baby's brain, organs and muscles are developing.

- **Folate:** to reduce the risk of neural rube defects. Green leafy vegetables, spinach, asparagus, peas, lentils, fortified grains (whole grain bread and cereals).
- **Iron:** to meet the demands of extra blood volume. Lean red meat, dates, black-eyed peas, spirulina, bok choy, sardines, spinach.
- **Omega-3:** DHA (Docosahexaenoic Acid) for the brain. Oily fish such as salmon, tuna, sardines, mackerel and trevally.

- **Iodine:** to balance your hormones at this demanding time, and support the metabolism and growth of your baby. Kelp, spirulina, dulse, cranberries, apricots, potatoes.
- **Zinc:** every cell of the body (yours and baby's) needs zinc to do its job. Avocado, raspberries, oily fish, peas, asparagus, pumpkin seeds.

2nd Trimester: This is the time for growth! The organs begin to work, eyes and ears develop and cartilage forms into bones.

- **Calcium:** for bone, muscle and nerve health. Dates, dairy produce (yoghurt especially), oranges, almonds, sesame seeds, celery.
- **Vitamin D:** to lay the foundation for strong bones. Oily fish, e.g. salmon, tuna and sardines, eggs, fortified cereals.
- **Co-enzyme Q10:** to support circulation, nerves and heart. Red meat, herring, trout, broccoli, oranges, strawberries and peanuts.

3rd Trimester: Baby requires all the nutrients above – even more so now – as organs, nerves, brain and bones finalise their development. For Mum, increasing protein at this stage through fish, lean meat, nuts and seeds will help stabilise blood sugars, help boost energy and ensure healthy growth of the baby.

Supplements: If you struggle to include all the nutrients above, or have concerns that your diet may be lacking, supplements can help.

Appendix 9
Food and Symptom Diary

Keeping a food and symptom diary is a great way to record everything you eat and drink and your body's response. Whether you have a skin issue, digestive problems or even suffer with anxiety and depression, if there is a food culprit triggering your symptom(s), a food diary can highlight what it might be. One of my clients identified green tea as her enemy after she kept a 4-week food and symptom diary. Once she eliminated it, her health significantly improved.

Due to the ways our various antibodies respond when under attack, bear in mind that your 11 am banana may be the cause of your 3 pm headache. Don't worry, it's easy for a trained eye to spot connections like these, so if there's nothing immediately obvious jumping out at you, take your diary along to your nutritionist for discussion and advice.

The Food and Symptom Diary chart opposite is available as a free download on the 'Free Fact Sheets' page at: www.alisoncowell.com

Time	Type and Amount of Food	Cooking Method	Dressings, Sauces, Spreads, etc.	Drink	Gas, Bloating, Reflux, Nausea, Heartburn, Bowel Movements, etc.

About Me

I was born in Buckinghamshire to Scottish parents and I had a very happy childhood. When I was a child I decided I wanted to either be an actress or a housewife because both lifestyles appealed. I excitedly auditioned for a local production of the Sound of Music when I was 10, but a consolation Quality Street and a sympathetic pat on my head as I left told me that the stage was not my destination.

I met my husband Steve when I was 15 and we married in 1978. When my first son was born in 1979 I took a keen interest in health and nutrition because I wanted the best for my baby. When my second son was born in 1980 I made every effort to make sure my boys were as well fed as they could be, within the limited budget I had.

I worked for the UK government between 1975 and 2005. In the early 2000s I was diagnosed with ulcerative colitis but I knew that I could help myself by focusing on the right nutrition. I studied and gained qualifications in both conventional and holistic nutrition. Happily, I have been in long-term remission ever since.

A move to New Zealand in 2005 provided the opportunity to open my health consultation business and I loved every second of my 13 years in such a stunning country. During that time, I saw over 10,000 individual clients with all manner of health issues. Apart from running my business, I presented an award-winning radio show; developed a health collaborative consisting of a range of health practitioners; hosted two health expos a year, raising funds for local charities; collaborated with businesses to promote health messages to staff and published my first book.

I returned to the UK in 2018 to be with my family. My parents are in their 90s and I have been blessed with gorgeous grandchildren. I decided to focus on speaking engagements on my return, but the pandemic put paid to that! Now, I still offer personal consultations and workshops, all online, and am delighted when I am invited to speak at various events.

Random facts about me:

- I am a qualified book keeper (I wanted to save money on accountancy fees)
- Just before my 40th birthday, I appeared on the BBC's 'National Lottery Dreamworld' . I wore a massive ballgown designed by Isabell Kristensen and, escorted by a troupe of young dancers, I pranced down the stairs at The Natural History Museum into a sea of celebrities who were attending a charity event
- Talking of dresses, I won a competition and met David Emanuel who designed a beautiful (very '80s) dress, which I still have to this day
- I jumped out of a plane at 15,000 feet; the free-falling bit through a cloud was painful!
- I love giraffes.

Acknowledgements

Many thanks to Martin and Nicki Lampon of Tiger Media and publisher Sarah Houldcroft for their support, knowledge and expertise in helping with the production of this book. The time difference between New Zealand and the UK made for some early morning/late evening meetings!

Thank you to my lovely niece Nina Jervis (NinaTheWriter) for coming up with the title.

To every single one of the amazing clients I have seen; your trust in me, the sharing of your health concerns and, most importantly, your results, inspire and motivate me every day.

Last but not least, a final thank you to those amongst my family and friends for being as excited about this as I am!

Index

A

Acne 98–9
Alopecia 114–5
Angina 127
Anxiety 98
Asthma 130
Atrial fibrillation 127–8
Autoimmune diseases 136–40

B

B vitamins 39, 97, 167-9, 172
Bloating 65-6
Blood pressure 124–6, 148–9
Bowel 15–6
Bronchitis *see* Chronic obstructive pulmonary disease

C

Calcium 39, 80, 83,174-189, 191-5, 219
Cancer 91-3, 146–8
Cellulite 111
Cellulitis 111–3
Cholesterol 122–4, 152-3
Chromium 168
Chronic fatigue syndrome 141–5
Chronic obstructive pulmonary disease 130–1
Co-enzyme Q10 166–7
Colon, *see* Bowel
Constipation 71–2
COPD *see* Chronic obstructive pulmonary disease
Covid *see* Long Covid
Crohn's disease 63, 75, 138

D

Depression 95–8
Dermatitis 107
Diabetes 81–3, 97, 128, 159
Diarrhoea 72–4
Diverticular disease 74–5

E

Eczema 48, 102-3, 106–8
Emphysema *see* Chronic obstructive pulmonary disease
Endometriosis 86–7, 165
Evening primrose oil 165
Eyes 100–1

F

Fertility *see* Infertility
Fibromyalgia 141–2
FODMAPs 67–71

G

Gallbladder 18, 58-62
Gallstones 58–60, 62
Gluten 48
Goitre 78
Gout 119–20
Grave's disease 80–1, 138

H

Hashimoto's disease 80, 138
Hay fever 135
Heart attack 126
High blood pressure *see* Blood pressure
Hives *see* Urticaria

Hyperthyroidism 80–1, 204–5
Hypothyroidism 79–80, 157–8, 204–5

I
IBS *see* Irritable bowel syndrome
Infertility 88
Indigestion 58, 214
Insomnia 99
Intestines, *see* Bowel
Iron 38-39, 163, 172
Irritable bowel syndrome 62–4, 67
Itching *see* Rashes, Eczema, Dermatitis, Urticaria

K
Kidneys 19-21, 119

L
Lactose 48-49
Leg ulcers 113–4
Levothyroxine 157–8
Lichen sclerosus 110
Liver 17
Long Covid 144–5
Low blood pressure *see* Blood pressure
Lymphatic system 18, 134

M
Magnesium 35-6, 122, 142, 164-5
Melanoma 114
Menopause 89-91, 216
Metformin 159
Microbiome 27, 50–1
Migraines 94–5
Myalgic encephalomyelitis 142

O
Oesophagus 14, 40, 57
Omega-3 166
Osteoarthritis 117–8
Osteopenia 116–7
Osteoporosis 117

P
Pancreas 18-9
Parasites 77
Perimenopause *see* Menopause
Polycystic ovary syndrome 19, 84, 159
Pregnancy 132–3, 218–9
Pre-menstrual tension 83, 165
Probiotics 27–31
Prostate 91–3
Psoriasis 109, 138

R
Rashes 103–5
Reflux 56–7
Rheumatoid arthritis 118–9, 138
Rosacea 110

S
Selenium 148, 169
Short bowel syndrome 76
Sleep *see* Insomnia
Small intestinal bacterial overgrowth 67, 110
Spleen 18
Stomach 15
Stroke 128–9

T
Throat 14
Thyroid disorders 78–71
Tongue 14, 36–9

U

Ulcerative colitis 75, 138
Urticaria 107

V

Varicose veins 129
Vitamins 39, 163–4
Vitamin A 39, 100, 163, 169
Vitamin B 39, 121, 167–8
Vitamin B12 37, 39, 159, 168, 172
Vitamin C 39, 163
Vitamin D 39, 162–3, 169
Vitamin E 169

W

Warfarin 159

Z

Zinc 39, 165, 171-2